America's Best Cookbook
for
Kids with Diabetes

America's Best Cookbook *for* Kids with Diabetes

Colleen Bartley

Introduction by Doreen Yasui RD, CDE

Robert ROSE

For complete cataloguing information, see page 180.

Disclaimer
The recipes in this book have been carefully tested by our kitchen and our tasters. To the best of our knowledge, they are safe and nutritious for ordinary use and users. For those people with food or other allergies, or who have special food requirements or health issues, please read the suggested contents of each recipe carefully and determine whether or not they may create a problem for you. All recipes are used at the risk of the consumer.

We cannot be responsible for any hazards, loss or damage that may occur as a result of any recipe use.

For those with special needs, allergies, requirements or health problems, in the event of any doubt, please contact your medical adviser prior to the use of any recipe.

Design & Production: PageWave Graphics Inc.
Editor: Sue Sumeraj
Recipe Tester: Jennifer MacKenzie
Proofreader: Sheila Wawanash
Indexer: Gillian Watts
Photography: Mark T. Shapiro
Food Styling: Kate Bush
Props Styling: Charlene Erricson
Color Scans & Film: Rayment & Collins

Cover image: Chocolate Chip Cookies (see recipe, page 138)

The publisher and author wish to express their appreciation to the following supplier of props used in the food photography:

Gourmet Settings Inc.
245 West Beaver Creek Road, Unit 10
Richmond Hill, Ontario L4B 1L1
Tel: 1-800-551-2649
www.gourmetsettings.com

We acknowledge the financial support of the Government of Canada through the Book Publishing Industry Development Program (BPIDP) for our publishing activities.

Published by Robert Rose Inc.
120 Eglinton Avenue East, Suite 800, Toronto, Ontario, Canada M4P 1E2
Tel: (416) 322-6552 Fax: (416) 322-6936

Printed in Canada

1 2 3 4 5 6 7 8 9 FP 12 11 10 09 08 07 06 05

Contents

Introduction

IT IS ESTIMATED that there are presently over 20 million North Americans living with diabetes. Up to a third of these have not been diagnosed. Types 1 and 2 are the most common types of diabetes and make up about 10% and 90% respectively of those who have this condition. Individuals with type 1 are most often diagnosed during their young childhood, in their teen years or as young adults, whereas those with type 2 are usually diagnosed as adults over the age of 40. It is unfortunate and alarming to see an increasing number of children and teens being diagnosed with type 2 diabetes, as just 20 years ago this condition was rarely seen in children. Some researchers fear that of all babies born today, one out of three will someday have diabetes!

In treating diabetes, the goal is to keep blood glucose levels within the target range recommended by a doctor, dietitian or diabetes education center. To achieve the recommended levels, type 1 diabetes is managed with daily insulin injection or pump therapy, individualized meal patterns based on exchanges or carbohydrate counting, and exercise or physical activity. Type 2 diabetes is managed through well-balanced, nutritious eating habits, with carbohydrate foods spread throughout the day, along with regular physical activity and weight management. Medications such as an oral pill and/or insulin may be used.

In both cases, checking blood sugar and having blood sugar readings in the range recommended by a diabetes education center is the goal. The A1C blood test reflects the average blood sugar level over the past two to three months. An A1C result in the desired range can (but does not always) reflect optimal diabetes care.

The recipes in this cookbook have the carbohydrate, protein and fat listed to allow parents and their children with type 1 diabetes to choose foods that fit into their meal plan and thus help them have good blood sugar control. Because most of the recipes are low in sugar and fat, they can be enjoyed by the whole family, whether they are siblings, parents, grandparents or extended family members who want to eat healthier meals.

When children are still young, many families eat simple, child-friendly foods. All the recipes in this cookbook have been taste-tested by kids, as well as their parents, relatives and friends. They are suitable for people of all ages, whether they have diabetes or not. The dishes are tasty, nutritious and easy to make. Some of the recipes are so simple that a child can prepare them, while others require adult guidance. It is my belief that, when children and teens are encouraged to help in the kitchen and are involved in food preparation, they have more interest in nutrition, food balance and meal planning. They can also develop an interest in cooking — an excellent skill to have! If teens can fend for themselves in the kitchen, there's less need for parents to worry when it comes time for them to move out or go on to college.

Meal Planning for Diabetes

WHEN YOUR CHILD is diagnosed with diabetes, it is essential to consult with a dietitian, who will help you identify eating habits suitable for promoting good diabetes care. Your dietitian will help you create a meal plan for your child that is well balanced and adequate in nutrients and calories.

Carbohydrate Counting

In recent years, there has been a gradual shift in meal planning toward a method popularly called carbohydrate counting, or carb counting for short. This method involves knowing how much carbohydrate one eats. The food groups that contain carbohydrates are Starch, Fruit, Vegetables, Milk and Other Carbohydrates. (It's important to keep in mind that, even though the Meat & Meat Substitute and Fat groups have no carbohydrates, they do contribute calories. Therefore, care should be taken to eat them to meet the needs of normal growth and development. The Meat & Meat Substitute and Fat groups are not considered "free" foods.)

Carbohydrate counting can work in two ways:

1 Choose foods at each meal and snack that tally up to a preplanned number of grams of carbohydrate per day. In this way, your usual insulin dosage should handle the amount of carbohydrate eaten.

You and your dietitian may discuss what a typical eating pattern would be for the day, and then establish carbohydrate counts for each meal and snack. For example, at lunchtime, if you usually eat a sandwich, a medium-sized piece of fruit, 2 plain cookies and a cup of milk, your carb count for the meal would be about 72 grams.

How does this work? Use the food groups and the carbohydrate values assigned to the groups in the American Diabetes Association Exchange System to find the total.

Food	Food Group	Carb Value per Choice	Total Carbs
1 sandwich	2 Starch choices	15 g	30 g
2 cookies	1 Starch choice	15 g	15 g
1 medium apple	1 Fruit choice	15 g	15 g
1 cup milk	1 Milk choice	12 g	12 g
Total carb count at lunch			*72 g*

Even when you decide to eat a lunch that's quite different from your usual sandwich meal, as long as it adds up to about 72 grams, your usual insulin dosage will look after it.

2 Add up the carbs from all the carbohydrate-containing foods in the meal you plan to eat, and then use an insulin-to-carb ratio predetermined by your diabetes care team. This can work well if you take fast-acting insulin before that meal or if you are using an insulin pump. There are various resources available to help you add up the carbs. Many fast-food restaurants have a handout sheet with this information, most packaged products have a "Nutrition Facts" label, and many websites provide this information.

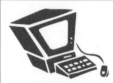 For a list of foods and their carb counts, check out the USDA's website: **www.nal.usda.gov/fnic/foodcomp**. Select "Reports by Single Nutrient" and then select "carbohydrate."

Nutritional Considerations When Carbohydrate Counting

As flexible and convenient as carb counting can be in blood sugar management with multiple daily injections and pump therapy, there are a couple of pitfalls to watch for and avoid:

1 The freedom to eat what and how much you wish may mean you eat more than you really need. This can mean unwanted weight gain.

2 Carb counting means paying attention to the carbohydrate-containing foods you eat, but this isn't all that is important when it comes to getting good nutrition or having optimal blood sugar levels. Will having a sugary drink or a plate of french fries with gravy that adds up to the usual lunch carb count really do the trick? What about getting enough milk, fruits, vegetables and protein foods? What about getting too much fat, or the wrong kinds of fat? These are all questions to think about beyond the basics of carb counting.

What Are Carbohydrates?

When we think of carbohydrates, **starch foods** such as cereals, potatoes, rice, pasta, and bread likely come to mind. Other starches are corn, popcorn, crackers, biscuits, croissants and grains such as barley, couscous and quinoa. But **sugars** and **fiber** are also carbohydrates. Starch and sugars both break down in digestion and end up as blood glucose or blood sugar. Carbohydrates supply approximately 4 calories per gram and should make up about half the total daily calories.

How Much Sugar Is Okay?

It is now accepted that, even when a person has diabetes, added sugar is not a bad thing when eaten in measured amounts. As a matter of fact, up to 10% of the total calories eaten in a day can come from added sugar. What this means is, if a person eats 1800 calories a day, 180 of these can be derived from added sugar, which works out to 45 grams of sugar. This translates in real food to 1 chewy trail-mix granola bar (13 g sugar), 1 lower-fat chocolate pudding (19 g sugar), and ¾ cup (175 mL) oatmeal crisp maple nut cereal (13 g sugar). It doesn't take much! Foods containing added sugar can be substituted for fruit or starch in the meal plan or can be used when a person taking insulin is more active than usual and chooses to have more carbohydrate to keep the blood sugar level normal. (Some people may prefer to compensate for activity by decreasing their insulin.)

Sugar can come in the form of granulated sugar, brown sugar, confectioner's (icing) sugar, honey, molasses and regular jam, jelly or syrup. The recipes in this cookbook use real sugar, but if you feel that the sugar or caloric content is too high, a sugar substitute can be used instead. If you are using Equal® (aspartame) or Splenda® (sucralose) in your baking, substitute an amount that's equivalent to the total sugar or to a portion of the sugar. Both of these products are made to have similar sweetness to sugar. Therefore, ½ cup (125 mL) of sugar can be substituted with ½ cup (125 mL) Equal or Splenda, which would reduce the carbohydrates by about 88 grams and the total calories by 337. Read the package directions carefully for instructions on how to use these sugar substitutes. Splenda, for example, is to be mixed in with the dry ingredients rather than blended in with the fat.

Many parents ask about the safety of sugar substitutes, especially aspartame, which is used most commonly in sugar-free beverages and in ready-to-eat, prepared and packaged products. Safety levels are set for various sweeteners based on body weight, and parents must keep in mind that children have smaller bodies and will therefore reach their safety level with a smaller amount of the sugar substitute. Talk to your dietitian about how much is safe for your child.

MEAL PLANNING FOR DIABETES

Another type of sugar substitute is the sugar alcohol used in products such as sugar-free chocolate bars, candies, chewing gum, syrups and fruit spreads. Examples of sugar alcohols are isomalt, lactitol, mannitol, maltitol, sorbitol and xylitol. Note that all except isomalt end with "-itol" — it will help you remember the names. Sweets with sugar alcohols should be limited, as large amounts can cause stomach upset, bloating and diarrhea.

Approximately 50% of total sugar alcohol turns into blood glucose. So, for carbohydrate counting, if a label tells you how much total sugar alcohol is present in the food, count it as half of the total. For example, if an ice cream bar contains 8 grams of sorbitol, only 4 grams would be used toward the carb count. Talk to your dietitian about how to read labels of foods with sugar alcohols.

Polydextrose, another carbohydrate commonly found in sugar-free, low-fat ice creams, is not broken down to sugar, does not affect blood sugar and does not need to be included in carbohydrate counting.

The ingredients in packaged food are listed in order of the amount in the package. If sugar is listed near the beginning of the list, then it is one of the main ingredients in that food. Watch for other words on the ingredient list that mean sugar, such as fructose, glucose-fructose, sucrose, maltose, lactose, honey, liquid sugar, invert sugar, liquid invert sugar, syrup, galactose, dextrose, dextrin, high-fructose corn syrup, corn syrup solids, molasses and raisin syrup.

Facts on Fiber

Dietary fiber is the part of a plant we can't digest; as a result, it is not considered to supply any calories or add to our blood sugar. But just because we don't digest fiber doesn't mean it's not an important nutrient. Researchers are letting us know that fiber is important in reducing the risk of colon cancer, lowering blood cholesterol and helping with bowel regularity.

There are two main types of fiber: soluble and insoluble. Both are good for you in different ways.

Soluble fiber is found in oat bran, oatmeal, legumes, apples and citrus fruits. This type of fiber forms a gel in the upper part of your intestine that traps cholesterol and slows down the absorption of sugar. This can help lower blood cholesterol and control blood sugar levels, so your blood sugar doesn't increase as quickly or have as large a peak after a meal.

Insoluble fiber is found in wheat bran and whole-grain breads and cereals, as well as in fruits and vegetables. This is the type of fiber that keeps you regular. If you're beginning to add more fiber to your diet, do it slowly, and remember to drink plenty of fluids to help prevent discomfort.

How Much Fiber Should I Eat?

Most people do not eat enough fiber, getting only about half of the recommended intake of 25 to 35 grams per day. Children need fiber too! Children and adults alike face health risks when they regularly eat fast foods, packaged foods and processed foods instead of making meals and snacks from scratch. Children older than two should eat enough fiber to equal their age plus 5 grams per day. For example, the daily fiber intake of a 10-year-old should be 15 grams per day.

MEAL PLANNING FOR DIABETES

How Can I Add More Dietary Fiber?

There are several ways you can add fiber to your diet:

- eat whole wheat, pumpernickel or multi-grain breads with your meals;
- eat 5 or more servings of vegetables and fruit daily;
- start your day with a high-fiber cereal, one that has at least 4 grams of fiber per serving;
- eat fresh fruit for dessert, and use it as a topping for yogurt or cereal;
- add nuts and seeds to a vegetarian stir-fry;
- where possible, leave the peel on vegetables (for example, potatoes and carrots);
- try some of the recipes in this book that include legumes;
- read package labels to find food products that have higher fiber sources (foods that claim to be "a source of fiber" must have at least 2.5 grams of fiber per serving and "a high source" at least 5.5 grams.)

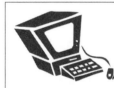 For a complete list of fiber-containing foods, see the USDA's website: **www.nal.usda.gov/fnic/foodcomp**. Select "Reports by Single Nutrient" and then select "total dietary fiber."

Label Reading for Carbohydrates

The "Nutrition Facts" table provides information on 13 nutrients, based on the serving size shown. It is important to keep the serving size in mind, since having a smaller or larger serving changes not only the nutrient content but — especially important in diabetes — the total carbohydrate content. The % Daily Value puts nutrients on a scale from 0% to 100% and tells you if there is a little or a lot of a nutrient in one serving of that packaged food. This value is based on a 2000-calorie intake.

All packaged food labels include amounts of total carbohydrate, dietary fiber and sugars. The dietary fiber and sugars amounts are indented under total carbohydrate, indicating they are part of the total grams of carbohydrate. To determine the amount of carbohydrate that really counts in raising blood sugar, grams of fiber must be subtracted from total grams of carbohydrate. The remaining amount is referred to as the amount of "available carbohydrate," which will convert into blood glucose.

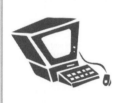

For examples of food labels and more details on how to read them, see the American Diabetes Association's website (**www.diabetes.org**) or the Food and Drug Administration's Center for Food Safety and Applied Nutrition website (**vm.cfsan.fda.gov/~dms/foodlab.html**).

Nutrition Claims on Labels

Manufacturers may or may not choose to put a nutrition claim on their food label. The food product must meet certain criteria set forth by the Food and Drug Administration to have a nutrition claim displayed on the package. In this way, consumers are assured that claims are credible and are consistent with current scientific and dietary recommendations.

A commonly misunderstood term is "no added sugar." It means there is no sugar *added* to the food. However, there may be sugar in the food to begin with. Don't be fooled by the claim on fruit juice that states "no added sugar": the natural sugar from the fruit is, of course, still there. This fruit juice can be used in regular meal planning or for treating low blood sugar, but it is not considered a sugar-free juice.

"Light" is a claim that is allowed on foods that are "reduced in fat" or "reduced in calories." "Light" can also be used to describe a feature of the food such as "light in color." If the word "light" is used on a food label, it must have a statement that explains what characteristic makes the food "light."

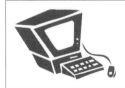 For more information on nutrition labeling, see the Food and Drug Administration's Center for Food Safety and Applied Nutrition website: **vm.cfsan.fda.gov/~dms/fdnewlab.html**.

Facts on Fat

Fat provides energy and is a carrier for important nutrients. Fat in our bodies insulates against cold and cushions the skin, bones and internal organs. Fat also makes food taste good. However, if we eat too much fat, or too much of the unhealthy fats, it can contribute to obesity, heart disease and type 2 diabetes. But remember, young children need fat as a source of calories to support adequate growth and development and should not be on strict "low-fat" diets.

Fats can be divided into two main types: saturated and unsaturated.

Saturated Fats

Saturated fats are commonly found in foods of animal origin and include items such as eggs, meat, butter, cheese, whole milk, 2% milk, 1% milk, sour cream, ice cream, lard and shortening. The plant fats palm oil, palm kernel oil and coconut oil are also high in saturated fats.

Although **trans fats** occur naturally in some foods, such as meat and milk, most are formed in the process of making a liquid oil into a solid fat, such as in the manufacturing of margarine or vegetable shortening. This process is called "hydrogenation." Trans fats are found in packaged foods and various snack foods such as cookies, crackers, biscuits, potato chips, breakfast waffles and cake mixes, as well as in hydrogenated margarines. Food manufacturers use hydrogenated fats or oils in packaged food to make the product more shelf-stable, so that it can stay fresh longer.

Because trans fats increase LDL cholesterol (or "bad" cholesterol), it is recommended to eat them as little as possible. At present, research has not clearly established how much we should try to limit our intake. But together, the saturated and manmade trans fat in our diet should make up less than 10% of our total daily calories.

Unsaturated Fats

These can be **monounsaturated** or **polyunsaturated fats**.

Monounsaturated fats are found in vegetable oils such as canola, olive and peanut, as well as in nuts and seeds, olives, avocados and non-hydrogenated soft tub margarines. These fats lower LDL cholesterol while maintaining HDL cholesterol (the "good" cholesterol) and are considered better choices over saturated or polyunsaturated fats.

Polyunsaturated fats include oils made from sunflower or safflower seeds, corn, soybeans, nuts and seeds. These are made up primarily of omega-6 fatty acids. The polyunsaturated omega-3 fats are found in fatty fish such as salmon, mackerel, trout, sardines, swordfish and Atlantic herring. Omega-3 fats are considered beneficial for a heart-healthy diet because they prevent stickiness and clotting of the blood. The American Diabetes Association recommends eating fish two to three times a week. The plant sources of omega-3 fats are flaxseeds, walnuts and their oils. It is difficult to get enough of this type of fat in our daily diet, especially if one is not fond of fish.

Fats in foods such as eggs, milk, cheese and cookies are often hidden. These fats are described as being "invisible," but they're there! The presence of fat in other sources, such as in butter, margarine, vegetable oil and salad dressing, is more obvious. Here are some words for fats and saturated fat you may see on a food-product ingredients list: glycerides, esters, tallow or beef fat, suet, cocoa butter, hydrogenated fats and oils, powdered whole milk solids, coconut or coconut oil.

Whatever the source or the type of fat, it is wise for most people to keep the total amount limited. The recommendation of the American Diabetes Association is that total fat be no more than 30% of total daily calories. *A reduced fat intake is not recommended for children.* Generally, the expected intake for children is approximately 30% to 35% of total daily calories.

Each gram of fat supplies approximately 9 calories, compared to about 4 calories per gram for both carbohydrate and protein. Each teaspoon (5 mL) of fat has approximately 5 grams of fat, and therefore about 45 calories. For a teenage boy who eats 2800 calories daily, this means his fat calories should be 840 (30% of total), which equals 93 grams fat. This equals 18 tsp (90 mL) of invisible and visible fat per day, of which no more than 6 tsp (30 mL) should come from saturated fats. For a younger child eating 1800 calories, the fat calories should be 540 (30% of the total), or 60 grams of fat. This equals 12 tsp (60 mL) of fat per day, of which no more than 4 tsp (20 mL) should come from saturated fat.

This may sound rather complicated, but with the help of a dietitian who will guide you in the selection of foods with different types of fats and appropriate portion sizes, you can soon be making healthy choices in your daily menu planning without doing all the math.

MEAL PLANNING FOR DIABETES

The Glycemic Index

The glycemic index (GI) is a scale that ranks carbohydrate-rich foods by how much they raise blood glucose levels compared to a standard food of glucose or white bread. The amount that the food increases blood sugar is called the "glycemic response." Foods that have a low GI are digested and absorbed more slowly than foods with a high GI, resulting in a lower glycemic response. Foods are described as having a GI that is low (<55), intermediate (55–70) or high (>70), where glucose is the reference standard and is given a value of 100.

The concept of GI challenged traditional views that "complex starches" require longer to digest and therefore affect blood sugar less than "simple sugars," and that these simple sugars should be avoided in the diabetic diet. Research has shown that the GI of table sugar is actually less than that of some starches, such as refined cereal or rice, which has been shown to have a very high GI. We now have evidence to support the idea that sugars and sweet treats used *in moderation* do not affect blood sugar any differently than many starches and can be used safely in a diabetic diet. Due to findings such as this, the terms "complex starch" and "simple sugar" are no longer used to describe types of carbohydrates in the diabetic diet, as they do not correctly reflect the effect on blood glucose.

Many factors play a role in lowering the glycemic response of foods. For example, foods high in soluble fiber, such as barley, rolled oats and kidney beans, have a lower GI than foods low in soluble fiber, such as cornflakes and instant rice. The presence of protein, fat, acids or sugars in food also lowers the glycemic response. (Keep in mind, though, that although high-sugar foods may have a lower GI than some starch foods, sugary foods can lack nutritional value). In addition, cooking and food preparation methods can make a difference:

- Al dente pasta has a lower GI than overcooked pasta.
- Whole boiled potatoes have a lower GI than mashed potatoes.

Because low-GI foods are digested and absorbed more slowly, blood sugar rises more slowly and at its peak is not as high as when foods with a higher GI value are eaten. Therefore, to prevent sharp rises and falls in blood sugar, it may be beneficial for the person with diabetes to choose foods of lower GI value more often.

However, the GI should not be used exclusively in deciding what to eat. Rather, it is important that you follow the guidelines and suggestions of your dietitian in getting all the food groups and nutrients considered healthful for a person with diabetes. The American Diabetes Association recommends that low-GI foods be included daily in the diet. But don't completely eliminate foods that have a high GI, as these foods can provide energy and nutrients.

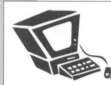

For more information on the glycemic index, see **www.diabetes.org**.

Vitamins and Minerals

Vitamins are essential nutrients. This means that your body needs these substances to function properly. Vitamins are needed only in small amounts and have no caloric value, but they help the body transform carbohydrate, protein and fat into energy.

There are two main types of vitamins. Fat-soluble vitamins — vitamins A, D, E and K — are found in and absorbed with the fats in our diet. Water-soluble vitamins include the B vitamins and vitamin C. Enjoy a wide variety of foods to meet your daily requirement of vitamins.

Minerals are naturally occurring inorganic substances required by the body. Calcium, phosphorous, magnesium, sodium, potassium, iodine, iron, zinc, manganese, chromium, copper, selenium and fluoride are all examples of minerals. Minerals are found in a wide variety of foods from each of the different food groups. Just as with vitamins, the most important thing is to remember to choose a wide variety of foods each day.

Children and teens who don't drink enough milk will find it difficult to get their daily requirement for calcium. Bone mineralization takes place primarily during the peak growth years. Therefore, it is essential for children and teens to have an adequate intake of milk or other sources of calcium, along with vitamin D, which the body needs in order to absorb calcium.

Vitamins and Minerals on the Nutrition Facts Table

Calcium, iron and vitamins A and C can now be found on all food labels. The amounts of these nutrients are expressed in percentages, so that you can see approximately how much of your daily requirement a serving of this food provides. Remember, though, that the percentages are based on a 2000-calorie diet, not the requirements for children.

What Are Antioxidants and Phytochemicals?

Foods deliver thousands of chemicals and substances other than the handful we call nutrients. As we learn more about the different compounds in foods and the role they may play in helping to prevent cancer and heart disease, the terminology that comes with the research can be confusing. Here are some words you might hear in the news.

Free radicals are unstable molecules that can damage the cells of the body. This damage is called **oxidative stress**. **Antioxidants** and **phytochemicals** are food compounds that help fight free radicals and protect the body. Examples of antioxidants are vitamins A, C and E and phytochemicals, all of which can be found in fruits and vegetables.

The best course of action is to eat a wide variety of fruits and vegetables and not to single out a particular nutrient that we think will be the magical answer. Research shows that it may be the combination and interaction of different chemicals that provides the body with maximum health benefits.

Get Moving!

All children and youth should be physically active, and especially if they have diabetes. Exercise is good for us, in many ways. It helps us feel energized, works the heart (which is also a muscle), decreases the risk of chronic disease (such as cardiovascular disease), and prevents the body's metabolism from slowing down. If you're not already active, start with small simple changes. Meet a friend for a walk or a bicycle ride instead of having another snack; take the stairs instead of the elevator; play a game of pickup basketball with your family; and work your way up from there.

Parents can play an important role by setting a good example: they must show their children that activity can be fun and get them involved in exercise programs. Children who find an activity they enjoy will be set on a path that will guide them for the rest of their lives.

Breakfasts

This recipe is good for breakfast, brunch or a light supper.

Variation

You can use egg substitute instead of whole eggs; ¼ cup (50 mL) egg substitute equals 2 whole eggs.

Puffy Ham and Cheese Bake

- *Preheat oven to 350°F (180°C)*
- *8-inch (2 L) square baking dish, sprayed with vegetable spray*

4	slices whole wheat bread	4
1 tbsp	soft margarine	15 mL
1 cup	shredded lower-fat Cheddar or Swiss cheese	250 mL
½ cup	diced cooked ham	125 mL
3	large eggs	3
1 cup	1% milk	250 mL
½ tsp	salt	2 mL
½ tsp	freshly ground black pepper	2 mL
½ tsp	Dijon mustard	2 mL

1. Cut the crusts off 3 slices of bread; set crusts aside. Spread both sides of bread with margarine. Cut diagonally in half to make triangles and stand them up around the edges of the baking dish

2. Cut the reserved crusts and the remaining slice of bread into ½-inch (1 cm) cubes and spread them on the bottom of the baking dish.

3. Sprinkle the shredded cheese and diced ham evenly over the bread cubes.

4. In a small bowl, beat eggs, milk, salt, pepper and mustard; pour over the ham and cheese.

5. Bake in preheated oven for 35 to 40 minutes, or until the egg is set and the top is puffy and golden. Serve immediately.

Exchanges Per Serving

1	Starch
4	Medium-Fat Meat

Nutrient Analysis Per Serving

Calories	390
Protein	32 g
Fat	21 g
Saturated fat	10 g
Carbohydrate	19 g
Fiber	2 g
Cholesterol	213 mg
Sodium	1133 mg

Dietitian's Message *For brunch, serve with a fresh fruit salad. For lunch or supper, add a green salad or cooked vegetables for additional vitamins, minerals and other phytonutrients.*

Mexican Scrambled Eggs

Here is an easy way to add excitement to ordinary scrambled eggs. Olé!

- Preheat oven to 350°F (180°C)
- Large nonstick skillet, sprayed with vegetable spray

3	large eggs	3
3	large egg whites	3
2 tbsp	1% milk	25 mL
½ tsp	salt	2 mL
¼ tsp	freshly ground black pepper	1 mL
½ cup	shredded lower-fat Cheddar cheese	125 mL
¼ cup	chopped green onions	50 mL
¼ cup	diced red or green bell peppers	50 mL
4	8-inch (20 cm) flour tortillas	4
¼ cup	salsa (optional)	50 mL

1. In a medium bowl, whisk together eggs, egg whites, milk, salt and pepper. Stir in cheese, green onions and red and green peppers.

2. Wrap the tortillas in foil and warm in preheated oven for 10 minutes.

3. Meanwhile, preheat skillet over medium heat. Pour in the egg mixture. Stir gently with a spatula and, as the egg sets, lift the cooked portions and allow the uncooked portions to flow underneath until all the egg is completely set.

4. Spoon eggs into the center of the warm tortillas. Fold the tortillas over and serve with salsa, if desired.

Dietitian's Message

It is well known that eggs are an excellent source of protein, but they also contribute an abundance of iron, vitamin A, and B vitamins such as B_{12}, folate, B_6 and B_2. The additional egg whites in this recipe provide more volume without adding more cholesterol or fat.

Tip
Learning to scramble eggs is a great cooking lesson for kids.

Variation
If you like spicy foods, substitute Monterey Jack with jalapeño peppers for the Cheddar cheese. Also try using different flavors of tortillas, such as tomato or cheese, but be aware that different tortillas will have a different nutrient analysis.

Exchanges Per Serving

1½ Starch

1½ Medium-Fat Meat

Nutrient Analysis Per Serving

Calories	232
Protein	15 g
Fat	9 g
Saturated fat	3 g
Carbohydrate	22 g
Fiber	1 g
Cholesterol	170 mg
Sodium	596 mg

Surprise Quick Quiche

Tip

When frying bacon,
plan on making more
than you need. Freeze
the extra in freezer
bags for up to 1 month
so it's ready for use
in recipes such as
this one.

Variations

Substitute shredded
Swiss cheese and add
a diced tomato and a
diced cooked potato.

To make a meatless
version, leave out
the bacon bits and
add 1 cup (250 mL)
cooked chopped
broccoli and/or
1 cup (250 mL) cooked
sliced mushrooms.

Exchanges
Per Serving

1	Starch
2½	Medium-Fat Meat

Nutrient Analysis
Per Serving

Calories	254
Protein	20 g
Fat	12 g
Saturated fat	6 g
Carbohydrate	15 g
Fiber	1 g
Cholesterol	184 mg
Sodium	297 mg

- Preheat oven to 400°F (200°C)
- 9-inch (23 cm) pie plate, sprayed with vegetable spray

3	large eggs	3
1½ cups	1% milk	375 mL
¼ cup	whole wheat flour	50 mL
2 tbsp	cornmeal	25 mL
3	green onions, chopped	3
1¼ cup	shredded lower-fat Cheddar cheese	300 mL
3 tbsp	cooked bacon bits	45 mL

1. In a blender or food processor, combine eggs, milk, flour and cornmeal. Blend for 30 seconds, until well blended.

2. In the prepared pie plate, gently toss green onions, shredded cheese and bacon bits. Pour the milk mixture over the cheese mixture.

3. Bake in preheated oven for 20 to 22 minutes, or until a knife inserted in the center comes out clean.

Dietitian's Message *If you include the vegetables in the variation, this dish contains four healthy food groups. (Or serve with a side salad.) It's simply amazing how the flour and cornmeal in the mixture end up making the bottom crust of this delicious and quick meal.*

Eggs in Cereal Nests

- Preheat oven to 425°F (220°C), if using
- Four ¾-cup (175 mL) custard cups or ramekins

1 tbsp	soft margarine	15 mL
2 cups	bran flakes cereal	500 mL
¾ cup	shredded lower-fat Cheddar cheese	175 mL
4	large eggs	4
	Salt and freshly ground black pepper	

1. In a microwave-safe medium bowl, microwave margarine, uncovered, on High for 20 to 30 seconds, or until melted. Stir in bran flakes and cheese.

2. Spoon the bran flake mixture into the custard cups, making a well in the center of each. Break an egg into the center of each cereal "nest" and sprinkle with salt and pepper to taste.

3. Cover the cups with aluminum foil and bake in preheated oven for 10 to 12 minutes, or until eggs are set.

TO COOK IN THE MICROWAVE

3. Poke each yolk with a toothpick or the point of a sharp knife and microwave all four custard cups at once, covered with wax paper, on High for about 3 minutes, or until eggs are almost set.

Bake these eggs in a microwave instead of a conventional oven. When cooking eggs in the microwave, always pierce the yolks first, or the pressure could cause the yolks to explode!

Tips

If you microwave the eggs one at a time rather than all at once, heat each for 45 to 50 seconds (depending on your microwave).

Try different brands of lower-fat cheese to decide what kind you like. Some taste milder than regular cheese, so you might prefer to use old cheese when you would normally use medium.

Exchanges Per Serving

1	Starch
1½	Medium-Fat Meat
1	Fat

Nutrient Analysis Per Serving

Calories	208
Protein	14 g
Fat	12 g
Saturated fat	4 g
Carbohydrate	14 g
Fiber	2 g
Cholesterol	227 mg
Sodium	329 mg

Use this batter as a base for the delicious recipes on pages 32–33, or follow the directions below to make basic pancakes or waffles.

Tip

Pancakes become tough if flipped more than once, so don't flip them before they are ready.

Pancake or Waffle Batter

2 cups	all-purpose flour	500 mL
1 tbsp	baking powder	15 mL
1 tbsp	granulated sugar	15 mL
½ tsp	salt	2 mL
½ cup	plain yogurt	125 mL
1 tsp	baking soda	5 mL
1	large egg	1
1½ cups	1% milk (approx.)	375 mL
2 tbsp	melted butter or margarine	25 mL
1 tsp	vanilla	5 mL

1. In a large bowl, combine flour, baking powder, sugar and salt.
2. Place yogurt in a measuring cup; stir in the baking soda and let it foam.
3. In a small bowl, whisk together egg, milk, melted butter and vanilla until blended.
4. Add the yogurt mixture and the milk mixture to the flour mixture and stir until blended. Mixture should be thick and slightly lumpy; thin the batter with more milk if it is too thick.

Dietitian's Message *Add fruits to the batter as suggested: they are bursting with flavor, sweetness, antioxidants and fiber. Substituting a portion of the flour with grains such as oats also ups the fiber content. Fiber, in addition to protein (in the egg white) and fat (in the butter or margarine), helps to lower the glycemic index of the pancakes and slows down the blood sugar rise after eating.*

Exchanges Per Serving

2½ Starch

½ Fat

Nutrient Analysis Per Serving

Calories	247
Protein	8 g
Fat	6 g
Saturated fat	3 g
Carbohydrate	39 g
Fiber	1 g
Cholesterol	49 mg
Sodium	564 mg

TO MAKE PANCAKES

Preheat skillet or griddle sprayed with vegetable spray over medium heat until medium-hot. Working in small batches so pancakes don't run together, pour ¼ cup (50 mL) pancake batter for each pancake into the hot pan, leaving ½ inch (1 cm) between. When bubbles on the surface of the pancakes start to pop and the edges are golden, turn the pancakes and cook the other side for 1½ to 2 minutes, or until golden.

TO MAKE WAFFLES

Following the waffle iron instructions, cook waffles in preheated nonstick waffle iron for 4 to 5 minutes, or until steaming stops.

Variations

Add any of the following to the batter: 1 cup (250 mL) blueberries, cranberries, sliced fresh peaches or sliced bananas.

Substitute oat bran, rolled oats, whole wheat flour or cornmeal for ½ cup (125 mL) of the flour.

Turn ordinary pancakes into real kid-pleasers!

Teddy Bear Pancakes

- *Large nonstick skillet or griddle, sprayed with vegetable spray*

3 cups	Pancake or Waffle Batter (see recipe, page 30)	750 mL
	Raisins	
	Calorie-reduced pancake syrup (optional)	

1. Mix the batter according to the directions on page 30. Preheat skillet until medium-hot.

2. To form a teddy bear: Working in small batches so pancakes don't run together, pour ⅓ cup (75 mL) batter for the bear's body into the hot pan, then spoon on 2 tbsp (25 mL) for the head, and 1 tsp (5 mL) each for the ears, arms and legs; overlap the circles so they stick together.

3. Cook until the bubbles on the surface begin to pop and the edges are golden. Carefully flip and cook the other side until golden.

4. Decorate with raisins for eyes and noses. Serve with calorie-reduced pancake syrup, if desired.

Exchanges Per Serving

2½ Starch

½ Fat

Nutrient Analysis Per Serving

Calories	247
Protein	8 g
Fat	6 g
Saturated fat	3 g
Carbohydrate	39 g
Fiber	1 g
Cholesterol	49 mg
Sodium	564 mg

Eggs in Cereal Nests (page 29) ▶

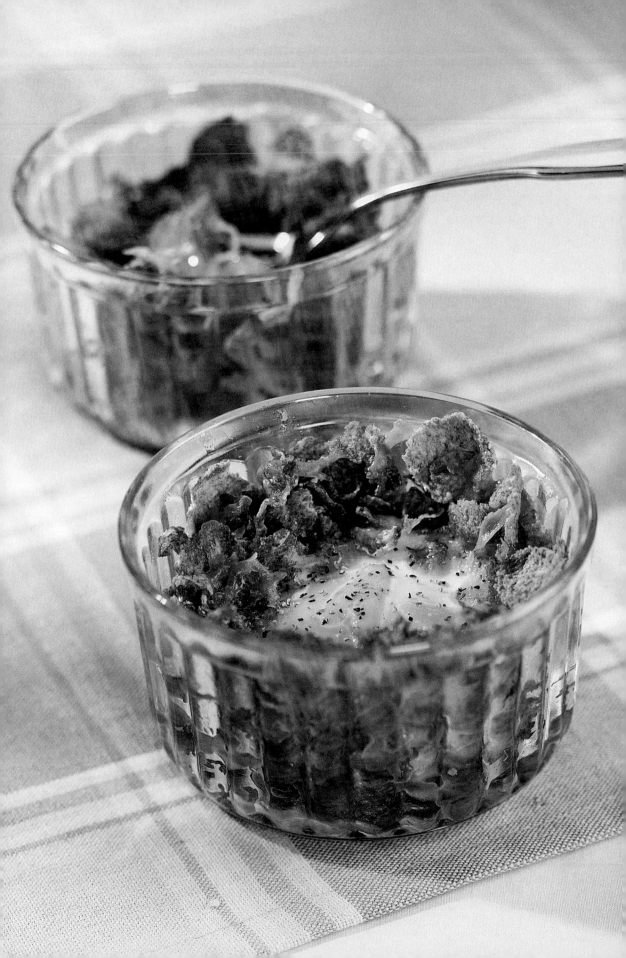

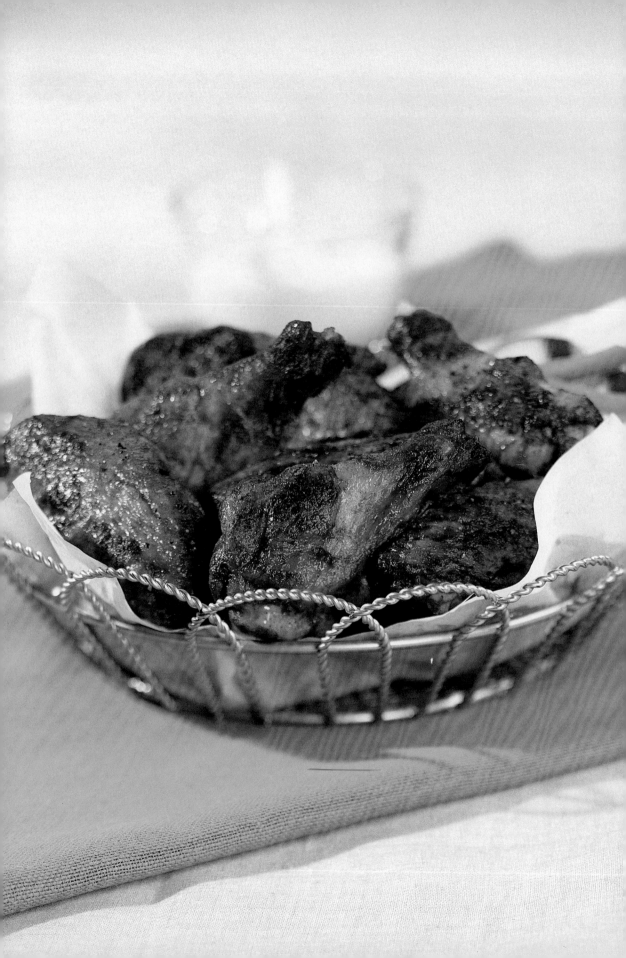

Happy Face Pancakes

- *Large nonstick skillet or griddle, sprayed with vegetable spray*

3 cups	Pancake or Waffle Batter (see recipe, page 30)	750 mL
½ tsp	ground cinnamon	2 mL
	Calorie-reduced pancake syrup (optional)	

1. Mix the batter according to the directions on page 30. Combine ⅓ cup (75 mL) of the batter with cinnamon. Preheat skillet until medium-hot.

2. Working in small batches so pancakes don't run together, drizzle cinnamon batter into the hot pan in the shape of eyes, nose, and mouth. Cook for 1 minute.

3. Pour 3 tbsp (45 mL) plain batter over each "face." Cook until the bubbles on the surface begin to pop and the edges are golden. Flip and cook the other side until golden.

4. Serve with calorie-reduced pancake syrup, if desired.

Variation

You can buy forms to make pancakes into different shapes at kitchen specialty stores, or you can use large metal cookie cutters to make Christmas tree, star or heart shapes. Spray the cookie cutter with vegetable spray and place it onto the hot grill. Pour the batter slowly and carefully into the cookie cutter; when the pancake begins to set, remove the cookie cutter. Use oven mitts, because the cookie cutter will be hot!

Exchanges Per Serving

2½ Starch

½ Fat

Nutrient Analysis Per Serving

Calories	247
Protein	8 g
Fat	6 g
Saturated fat	3 g
Carbohydrate	39 g
Fiber	1 g
Cholesterol	49 mg
Sodium	564 mg

◀ Buffalo Wings (page 66)

Pancake Banana Splits

Pancake banana splits are a great treat to surprise kids with after a slumber party!

Tip

When you are making pancakes using the batter recipe on page 30, you can make extra and freeze them in an airtight container with waxed paper separating the layers for up to 2 months. When ready to use, simply pop them into the toaster and then garnish with the sundae toppings.

Variation

Omit strawberries and top with crushed pineapple or fresh or frozen raspberries.

- *Large nonstick skillet or griddle, sprayed with vegetable spray*

1 1/2 cups	complete buttermilk pancake mix	375 mL
1 1/4 cups	water	300 mL
3	medium bananas, cut in half and sliced lengthways	3
1 1/2 cups	strawberry-flavored frozen yogurt	375 mL
1 1/2 cups	sliced strawberries	375 mL
1/3 cup	calorie-reduced strawberry or chocolate sundae topping (optional)	75 mL

1. Mix the batter according to the directions on the package. Preheat skillet until medium-hot.

2. Working in small batches so pancakes don't run together, pour 3 tbsp (45 mL) pancake batter for each pancake into the hot pan.

3. Cook until the bubbles on the surface begin to pop and the edges are golden. Carefully flip and cook the other side until golden.

4. To serve, overlap 2 pancakes on each plate. Place 1/2 banana on each serving. Top each with 1/4 cup (50 mL) frozen yogurt and 1/4 cup (50 mL) strawberries. Drizzle with 1 tbsp (15 mL) sundae topping, if using.

Exchanges Per Serving

2	Starch
1	Fruit
1/2	Fat

Nutrient Analysis Per Serving

Calories	264
Protein	6 g
Fat	5 g
Saturated fat	2 g
Carbohydrate	51 g
Fiber	3 g
Cholesterol	12 mg
Sodium	404 mg

Apple Oat Pancakes

MAKES 8 SERVINGS
(2 pancakes and
2 tbsp/25 mL apple
syrup per serving)

- *Large nonstick skillet or griddle, sprayed with vegetable spray*

⅓ cup	quick-cooking rolled oats	75 mL
2 cups	complete buttermilk pancake mix	500 mL
½ cup	grated apple	125 mL
2 tbsp	granulated sugar	25 mL
½ tsp	ground cinnamon	2 mL

Apple Syrup

| ¾ cup | unsweetened applesauce | 175 mL |
| ¼ cup | calorie-reduced pancake syrup | 50 mL |

Boost the nutrition and flavor of a pancake mix by adding oats and apple.

Tip
For very light pancakes, substitute club soda for the usual liquid in the batter.

I. In a medium bowl, combine 2 cups (500 mL) water and oats. Let stand for 5 minutes.

2. Add pancake mix, grated apple, sugar, and cinnamon to the oats. Stir just until mixed. Preheat skillet until medium-hot.

3. Working in small batches so pancakes don't run together, pour ¼ cup (50 mL) batter for each pancake into the hot pan. Cook until the edges look crisp and bubbles begin to break on the surface. Flip and cook the other side until golden.

4. *Meanwhile, prepare the apple syrup:* In a small saucepan, combine the applesauce and syrup. Heat over low heat until warm. Serve with the pancakes.

Dietitian's Message *Serve with Homemade Turkey Sausage (see recipe, page 39) as your protein choice for a hearty harvest breakfast.*

Exchanges Per Serving

| 2 | Starch |
| ½ | Other Carbohydrate |

Nutrient Analysis Per Serving

Calories	181
Protein	4 g
Fat	2 g
Saturated fat	0 g
Carbohydrate	37 g
Fiber	2 g
Cholesterol	7 mg
Sodium	395 mg

Protein Plus Pancakes

These pancakes can be frozen and reheated, which makes them very convenient on an active day.

Tips

To freeze: Layer in an airtight container with waxed paper separating the layers for up to 2 months.

To reheat: Preheat oven to 350°F (180°C). Place frozen pancakes in a single layer on a baking sheet and bake for 15 minutes.

- *Large nonstick skillet or griddle, sprayed with vegetable spray*

4	large eggs	4
I cup	1% cottage cheese	250 mL
1/3 cup	all-purpose flour	75 mL
3 tsp	vegetable oil, divided	15 mL
1/2 tsp	salt	2 mL

1. In a medium bowl, beat eggs with a whisk or a wooden spoon. Stir in cottage cheese, flour, 2 tsp (10 mL) vegetable oil and salt.

2. In skillet, heat the remaining 1 tsp (5 mL) oil. Spoon in batter in 4 mounds (cook 4 at a time), leaving 1 inch (2.5 cm) between each mound. Cook until edges turn golden; flip and cook the other side until golden brown.

Dietitian's Message *Serve these pancakes with sliced bananas and calorie-reduced pancake syrup to add carbohydrates to this meal.*

Exchanges
Per Serving

1/2	Starch
2	Medium-Fat Meat

Nutrient Analysis
Per Serving

Calories	185
Protein	15 g
Fat	9 g
Saturated fat	2 g
Carbohydrate	10 g
Fiber	0 g
Cholesterol	218 mg
Sodium	559 mg

Chocolate and Strawberry Waffles

It won't be hard to convince reluctant breakfast eaters to dig in when you serve these waffles! They look like dessert and taste delicious.

- Preheated waffle iron with a nonstick surface

2 cups	complete pancake and waffle mix	500 mL
1/4 cup	unsweetened cocoa powder, sifted	50 mL
1/4 cup	granulated sugar	50 mL
3 cups	sliced strawberries (about 2 pints)	750 mL
1 1/2 cups	lower-fat non-dairy whipped topping	375 mL
6	whole strawberries for garnish	6

1. In a medium bowl, combine waffle mix, cocoa and sugar. Mix well. Add 1 1/2 cups (375 mL) water and stir just until blended.

2. Following the waffle iron instructions, cook waffles in preheated waffle iron for 4 to 5 minutes, or until steaming stops.

3. Serve topped with sliced strawberries and whipped topping. Garnish each serving with a whole berry.

Dietitian's Message *There are many prepackaged pancake mixes on the market. Look for mixes that are low in fat and can be made with only the addition of water. Even a young teen can whip up these delicious waffles.*

Tip
When making waffles, make an extra batch for a quick breakfast another day. Cook the waffles, cool, and then freeze in a resealable plastic bag for up to 2 months. To reheat, pop them into the toaster and garnish with berries and whipped topping.

Exchanges Per Serving

2	Starch
1	Other Carbohydrate
1/2	Fat

Nutrient Analysis Per Serving

Calories	233
Protein	6 g
Fat	4 g
Saturated fat	1 g
Carbohydrate	46 g
Fiber	3 g
Cholesterol	15 mg
Sodium	514 mg

This is a great recipe for a special breakfast because it can be prepared the night before.

Tip

Day-old bread (French, Italian or sourdough) works better than fresh bread in this recipe.

Variation

Substitute other seasonal berries, such as raspberries, blackberries or blueberries, for the strawberries.

Exchanges Per Serving

1 ½ Starch

⅓ Fruit

½ Fat

Nutrient Analysis Per Serving

Calories	181
Protein	6 g
Fat	4 g
Saturated fat	2 g
Carbohydrate	30 g
Fiber	2 g
Cholesterol	81 mg
Sodium	352 mg

Crunchy French Toast

- *Rimmed baking sheet, sprayed with vegetable spray*

3	large eggs	3
⅓ cup	1% milk	75 mL
1 tbsp	granulated sugar	15 mL
½ tsp	vanilla	2 mL
¼ tsp	salt	1 mL
1 cup	corn flakes cereal	250 mL
8	slices French bread, cut on the diagonal ½ inch (1 cm) thick	8
2 cups	sliced fresh strawberries	500 mL
½ cup	lower-fat non-dairy whipped topping	125 mL

1. In a shallow bowl, whisk together eggs, milk, sugar, vanilla and salt; mix well.

2. Place corn flakes between 2 sheets of waxed paper, and crush into coarse crumbs with a rolling pin.

3. Dip bread into egg mixture and turn, letting it absorb liquid on both sides. Arrange the dipped bread in a single layer on the prepared baking sheet. Pour any remaining egg mixture over top. Sprinkle bread with cereal crumbs, pressing gently so that the crumbs adhere to the bread. Cover with plastic wrap and refrigerate for at least 6 hours but preferably overnight.

4. Preheat oven to 425°F (220°C). Remove plastic wrap and bake French toast, uncovered, in preheated oven for 20 to 25 minutes, or until knife inserted in the center comes out clean. Remove from oven.

5. Preheat the broiler and position the oven rack 6 to 7 inches (15 to 18 cm) from the element. Place French toast under the broiler and broil for 4 to 5 minutes, or until cereal topping is crispy and golden brown.

6. Serve topped with strawberries and whipped topping.

Dietitian's Message *Strawberries add a healthy dose of fiber and vitamin C, which are two nutrients our body needs daily. When they're not in season, use frozen unsweetened strawberries.*

Homemade Turkey Sausage

Homemade sausage is healthy, tasty and easy to make.

- *Large nonstick skillet, sprayed with vegetable spray*

3 tbsp	quick-cooking rolled oats	45 mL
2 tbsp	minced onion	25 mL
2 tsp	dried parsley	10 mL
I tsp	salt	5 mL
½ tsp	freshly ground black pepper	2 mL
½ tsp	dried sage	2 mL
¼ tsp	ground cloves	I mL
¼ tsp	ground nutmeg	I mL
I	egg white	I
8 oz	lean ground turkey	250 g

1. In a small bowl, combine oats, onion, parsley, salt, pepper, sage, cloves and nutmeg.

2. In a medium bowl, beat egg white with a fork. Add turkey and oats mixture; mix well. Shape into 8 patties about ½ inch (1 cm) thick.

3. Preheat skillet over medium heat. Place patties in preheated pan and cook for 5 minutes. Flip and continue cooking for 5 to 7 minutes, or until no longer pink inside.

> **Dietitian's Message** *This lower-fat sausage can be used as a pizza topping or to accompany another dish. For example, serve with Apple Oat Pancakes (see recipe, page 35).*

Tip

Raw poultry can be a host for salmonella bacteria. Wash your hands before and after handling poultry, and use hot, soapy water to clean your cutting board, knife, counter and anything else the raw poultry touched.

Variation

Add 2 tbsp (25 mL) diced sun-dried tomatoes in with the oat mixture. As kids get older and more adventurous in their eating, try adding more sophisticated ingredients to basic recipes.

Exchanges Per Serving

2	Very Lean Meat

Nutrient Analysis Per Serving

Calories	94
Protein	14 g
Fat	2 g
Saturated fat	I g
Carbohydrate	4 g
Fiber	I g
Cholesterol	37 mg
Sodium	600 mg

This convenient hot oatmeal can be prepared the night before and baked in the morning. It is like having a warm oatmeal cookie for breakfast!

Tip

Leftover squares can be individually wrapped and refrigerated for up to 2 days. Warm as needed in the microwave on High for 1 to 1½ minutes.

Variation

Substitute fresh seasonal fruit for the raisins. Blackberries, blueberries, raspberries, sliced apples and peaches are all tasty substitutes.

Exchanges Per Serving

1	Starch
½	Fruit
½	Fat

Nutrient Analysis Per Serving

Calories	147
Protein	4 g
Fat	4 g
Saturated fat	2 g
Carbohydrate	25 g
Fiber	2 g
Cholesterol	41 mg
Sodium	165 mg

Baked Apple-Raisin Oatmeal

- 13- by 9-inch (3 L) baking pan, sprayed with vegetable spray

2	large eggs	2
1½ cups	unsweetened apple juice	375 mL
2 cups	quick-cooking rolled oats	500 mL
¼ cup	packed brown sugar	50 mL
2 tsp	baking powder	10 mL
1 tsp	ground cinnamon	5 mL
½ tsp	ground nutmeg	2 mL
½ tsp	salt	2 mL
½ cup	raisins	125 mL
2 tbsp	melted butter or margarine	25 mL
	Milk or yogurt (optional)	

1. In a large bowl, whisk together eggs and apple juice until well blended. Add oats, brown sugar, baking powder, cinnamon, nutmeg and salt and mix well. Stir in raisins and melted butter.

2. Pour into prepared baking dish and cover tightly with plastic wrap. Refrigerate for at least 3 hours or overnight.

3. Preheat oven to 350°F (180°C). Uncover the baking dish and bake in preheated oven for 45 minutes, until golden brown. Let cool for 10 minutes.

4. Cut into 12 squares and serve with milk or yogurt, if desired.

Dietitian's Message *Although the goal for healthy eating is a well-balanced daily food intake, breakfast is considered the single most important meal of the day. The word itself reminds us that with this meal we are literally "breaking our fast" from the evening before. Eating a healthy breakfast, such as oatmeal, gives us a good start on our energy and nutrients for the day.*

Fruity Granola

- *Preheat oven to 350°F (180°C)*
- *Rimmed baking sheet, sprayed with vegetable spray*
- *9-inch (2.5 L) square baking pan*

2½ cups	quick-cooking rolled oats	625 mL
¾ cup	wheat germ	175 mL
⅓ cup	slivered almonds	75 mL
⅓ cup	liquid honey	75 mL
1 tbsp	vegetable oil	15 mL
1 tsp	ground cinnamon	5 mL
¼ tsp	salt	1 mL
½ cup	raisins	125 mL
½ cup	chopped dried apricots	125 mL
½ cup	dried cherries, bananas or cranberries	125 mL
⅓ cup	chopped pitted dates	75 mL
¼ cup	sunflower seeds (without shells)	50 mL

It's great to have homemade granola on hand. Enjoy it for breakfast with yogurt or milk, or use it in a variety of recipes, such as dessert bars and Baked Apples with Granola (see recipe, page 172).

1. In a large bowl, combine oats, wheat germ, almonds, honey, oil, 1 tbsp (15 mL) water, cinnamon and salt. Spread mixture on prepared baking sheet.

2. Bake in preheated oven for 15 minutes, stirring several times, until dark golden. Using an oiled spatula, immediately pack the hot mixture into square baking pan and let cool to room temperature.

3. When mixture is cool, transfer back to the large bowl and break into pea-sized pieces. Stir in raisins, apricots, cherries, dates and sunflower seeds. Store at room temperature in an airtight container for up to 2 weeks.

Dietitian's Message *Like most granola, this is packed with energy. The rolled oats and fruit make this high in carbohydrate, but with a good amount of fiber. Take care with the serving size to avoid getting too much carbohydrate. Serve with plain yogurt for more protein.*

Exchanges Per Serving

1	Starch
1	Other Carbohydrate
½	High-Fat Meat
1	Fat

Nutrient Analysis Per Serving

Calories	235
Protein	6 g
Fat	8 g
Saturated fat	2 g
Carbohydrate	37 g
Fiber	5 g
Cholesterol	0 mg
Sodium	49 mg

Breakfast Quesadillas

Traditionally, quesadillas are fried, but these are oven-baked, resulting in a much lower fat content. But they still have lots of flavor!

Tip

This recipe calls for homemade turkey sausage and salsa, but store-bought can be substituted. Buy lower-fat turkey, chicken or Italian sausages and remove the casings before cooking them.

Variation

Turn up the heat on these quesadillas! If you like spicy Mexican food, substitute Monterey Jack cheese with jalapeño peppers for the mozzarella and use a spicy salsa.

Exchanges Per Serving

1½ Starch

1   Medium-Fat Meat

Nutrient Analysis Per Serving

Calories	190
Protein	12 g
Fat	6 g
Saturated fat	2 g
Carbohydrate	23 g
Fiber	2 g
Cholesterol	22 mg
Sodium	467 mg

- Preheat oven to 400°F (200°C)
- Large nonstick skillet, sprayed with vegetable spray
- Baking sheet, sprayed with vegetable spray

	Homemade Turkey Sausage mixture (see recipe, page 39)	
6	8-inch (20 cm) flour tortillas	6
⅓ cup	salsa (store-bought or see recipe, page 58)	75 mL
¾ cup	shredded part-skim mozzarella cheese	175 mL
⅓ cup	chopped green onions	75 mL
	Additional salsa (optional)	

1. Prepare the sausage mixture following the instructions on page 39, but do not form the mixture into patties.

2. Preheat skillet over medium heat. Add the sausage mixture and cook, stirring frequently, for 6 to 7 minutes, or until crumbly and no longer pink. Set aside.

3. Place 3 tortillas on prepared baking sheet. Spread each with ⅓ of the salsa. Spoon ⅓ of the cooked turkey sausage evenly onto each tortilla. Sprinkle each with ¼ cup (50 mL) shredded cheese and ⅓ of the green onions. Top with the remaining tortillas.

4. Bake in preheated oven for 8 minutes, or until cheese is melted and edges begin to crisp.

5. Cut each quesadilla in half and serve with additional salsa, if desired.

Beverages

Keep a supply of frozen bananas on hand to make power milk shakes for breakfast!

Tip

When your bananas become too ripe, freeze them to make smoothies. They don't even have to be peeled! Just toss them in the freezer whole, and thaw slightly to remove the peel easily just before using. Don't thaw them too much, though — use them frozen for a good milk shake consistency.

Exchanges Per Serving

1	Fruit
1	Reduced-Fat Milk
$1/2$	Other Carbohydrate
$1/2$	Medium-Fat Meat

Nutrient Analysis Per Serving

Calories	238
Protein	12 g
Fat	3 g
Saturated fat	1 g
Carbohydrate	44 g
Fiber	5 g
Cholesterol	6 mg
Sodium	108 mg

Blender Breakfast Blast

- *Blender or food processor*

1	banana, fresh or frozen, sliced	1
1 cup	frozen sliced strawberries	250 mL
1 cup	1% milk	250 mL
$1/2$ cup	plain yogurt	125 mL
$1/4$ cup	wheat germ	50 mL
2 tsp	liquid honey (optional)	10 mL

1. In blender, combine banana, strawberries, milk, yogurt and wheat germ. Blend for 1 to 2 minutes, or until smooth. Sweeten with honey, if desired.

Dietitian's Message *When you don't feel like eating breakfast, have a blast! A Blender Breakfast Blast, that is. With milk, yogurt, fruit and wheat germ, it's full of nutrients: protein, calcium, vitamins A, B, C and E, carbohydrate and fiber. It's an awesome way to start the day!*

Peach Melba Smoothie

- *Blender or food processor*

1	peach, pitted and chopped	1
1½ cups	soy milk	375 mL
1 cup	frozen raspberries	250 mL
½ cup	vanilla-flavored frozen yogurt	125 mL

1. In blender, combine peach, soy milk, raspberries and frozen yogurt. Blend for 1 to 2 minutes, or until smooth. Serve immediately.

Dietitian's Message

When choosing soy milk, check the label for the amount of carbohydrate per serving. Depending on the brand and flavor chosen, the carbohydrate can vary a lot. For example, one brand of vanilla-flavored soy milk has 9.4 g carbohydrate per 1-cup (250 mL) serving; another has 26 g. This can make quite a difference in the blood glucose response. Also, most flavored soy milks (Chocolate, Mocha, Strawberry, Soyaccino) have a higher sugar content than the original (plain) flavor. Check to make sure the soy milk you choose is "fortified." This means nutrients are added, such as calcium and vitamins D, B_{12} and B_2, and other vitamins and minerals normally present in or added to cow's milk.

MAKES 2 SERVINGS

Healthy smoothies are a great pick-me-up at any time of the day!

Variation

Use regular 1% milk instead of soy milk or, for a dairy-free smoothie, substitute frozen soy beverage for the frozen yogurt.

Exchanges Per Serving

½	Starch
½	Other Carbohydrate
1	Medium-Fat Meat

Nutrient Analysis Per Serving

Calories	165
Protein	7 g
Fat	6 g
Saturated fat	2 g
Carbohydrate	24 g
Fiber	5 g
Cholesterol	1 mg
Sodium	53 mg

The flavor combinations for smoothies are endless. This one combines the kid-approved flavors of peanut butter, banana and strawberries in a energizing treat!

Tip

To make a smoothie for one, halve the ingredients and use an "electric wand" (immersion/hand-held blender) instead of a regular blender for easy cleanup.

Variation

Substitute chocolate milk or chocolate-flavored soy milk for the soy milk in this smoothie.

Exchanges Per Serving

1	Fruit
1/2	Reduced-Fat Milk
1/2	Other Carbohydrate
1	High-Fat Meat
1	Fat

Nutrient Analysis Per Serving

Calories	292
Protein	12 g
Fat	13 g
Saturated fat	2 g
Carbohydrate	38 g
Fiber	5 g
Cholesterol	0 mg
Sodium	107 mg

Peanut Butter and Banana Smoothie

- *Blender or food processor*

1	frozen banana, sliced	1
1 1/2 cups	soy milk	375 mL
1 cup	frozen sliced strawberries	250 mL
2 tbsp	peanut butter	25 mL

1. In blender, combine banana, soy milk, strawberries and peanut butter. Blend for 1 to 2 minutes, or until smooth. Serve immediately.

> **Dietitian's Message** *Soy milk makes a healthy addition to your diet because it's an additional source of phytochemicals. It's a good idea to use soy milk in smoothies because mixing it with other ingredients masks the slightly unusual taste. You can substitute 1% milk for soy milk in any of these smoothies.*

Frosty Strawberry Shake

Homemade milk shakes are an easy and satisfying treat.

- Blender or food processor

½ cup	boiling water	125 mL
1	package (⅓ oz/10 g) no-sugar-added strawberry-flavored gelatin	1
2 cups	vanilla ice cream	500 mL
1 cup	1% milk	250 mL
½ cup	ice cubes, crushed	125 mL

1. Pour boiling water into the blender. Add gelatin powder and blend for 1 minute. Keep the blender running and add ice cream by large spoonfuls through hole in lid.

2. Turn off the blender; add milk and ice. Blend for another 30 seconds, or until smooth and thick. Serve immediately.

Exchanges Per Serving

1	Other Carbohydrate
1	Medium-Fat Meat
½	Fat

Nutrient Analysis Per Serving

Calories	167
Protein	6 g
Fat	8 g
Saturated fat	5 g
Carbohydrate	19 g
Fiber	0 g
Cholesterol	31 mg
Sodium	143 mg

This is a cool and delicious addition to your daily fruit servings when fresh peaches are in season.

Tip

You can make this recipe with all fresh fruit, but using some frozen results in a thicker "milk shake" consistency.

Variation

Substitute your favorite seasonal fruit or berries for the peach and banana.

Peachy Banana Shake

• *Blender or food processor*

1	ripe peach, peeled and sliced	1
1	frozen banana, sliced	1
⅔ cup	vanilla ice cream	150 mL

1. In blender, combine peach, banana and ice cream. Blend for 1 to 2 minutes, or until smooth. Serve immediately.

Dietitian's Message *Fruit shakes are a great way to increase your fruit and fiber intake for the day and can be a fun surprise to tempt a reluctant breakfast eater.*

Exchanges Per Serving

2	Fruit
1½	Other Carbohydrate
½	High-Fat Meat
1	Fat

Nutrient Analysis Per Serving

Calories	320
Protein	5 g
Fat	10 g
Saturated fat	6 g
Carbohydrate	57 g
Fiber	4 g
Cholesterol	39 mg
Sodium	72 mg

Lemon Iced Tea

- 16-cup (4 L) non-metal beverage container

12	orange pekoe tea bags (regular or decaffeinated)	12
6	lemon-flavored tea bags	6
6 cups	boiling water	1.5 L
1/2 cup	granulated sugar	125 mL
9 cups	cold water	2.25 L
2	lemons, sliced	2

1. Place orange pekoe and lemon tea bags in the beverage container. Pour in boiling water, cover and let steep for 10 minutes. Remove tea bags and stir in sugar. Let cool to room temperature, then stir in cold water.

2. Serve over ice, garnished with lemon slices.

Dietitian's Message *To make sugar-free iced tea, replace sugar with an amount of artificial sweetener that has the same sweetening power as 1/2 cup (125 mL) sugar. Using artificial sweetener will reduce the calories to 7 and the carbohydrate content to 3 g per serving.*

Iced tea is so refreshing on a hot summer day. Make it early and store it in the refrigerator so it is cold by the time you want to drink it.

Exchanges Per Serving

1/2 Other Carbohydrate

Nutrient Analysis Per Serving

Calories	30
Protein	0 g
Fat	0 g
Saturated fat	0 g
Carbohydrate	9 g
Fiber	0 g
Cholesterol	0 mg
Sodium	3 mg

For a refreshingly zingy change, try this spiced iced tea.

Spiced Iced Tea

- *16-cup (4 L) non-metal beverage container*

8	orange pekoe tea bags (regular or decaffeinated)	8
1 tsp	whole cloves	5 mL
4 cups	boiling water	1 L
½ cup	granulated sugar	125 mL
10 cups	cold water	2.5 L
2 cups	orange juice	500 mL
2	lemons, sliced	2

1. Place tea bags and cloves in the beverage container. Pour in boiling water, cover and let steep for 10 minutes. Remove tea bags and cloves with a slotted spoon and stir in sugar. Let cool to room temperature, then stir in cold water and orange juice.

2. Serve over ice, garnished with lemon slices.

Dietitian's Message *To reduce the calories and carbohydrate count, replace sugar with an amount of artificial sweetener that has the same sweetening power as ½ cup (125 mL) sugar. Using artificial sweetener will reduce the calories to 21 and the carbohydrate content to 6 g per serving.*

Exchanges Per Serving

½ Other Carbohydrate

Nutrient Analysis Per Serving

Calories	42
Protein	0 g
Fat	0 g
Saturated fat	0 g
Carbohydrate	11 g
Fiber	1 g
Cholesterol	0 mg
Sodium	3 mg

A Perfect Cup of Cocoa

1 cup	1% milk	250 mL
2 tsp	unsweetened cocoa powder, sifted	10 mL
2 tsp	granulated sugar	10 mL
1/2 tsp	ground cinnamon	2 mL
1/4 tsp	salt	1 mL
1/2 tsp	vanilla	2 mL
1/4 tsp	almond extract	1 mL
5	mini marshmallows	5

One of my daughters, Heather, is always trying to make the perfect cup of cocoa. This is her creation, inspired by a trip to Mexico, where the cocoa is divine.

Tips

For a Christmas treat, use a candy cane or a cinnamon stick for a stir stick.

Mexicans make their hot chocolate with chocolate tablets. You can duplicate the flavor more closely by using squares of semi-sweet chocolate, but be aware that this will change the nutrient analysis.

1. In a small saucepan, heat milk over medium-high heat for about 5 minutes, until hot but not boiling. (Or, in a microwave-safe measuring cup, microwave on High for 1 1/2 to 2 minutes (depending on your microwave). Do not overheat, or it will form a "skin.")

2. In a large mug, combine cocoa, sugar, cinnamon and salt. Add 2 tbsp (25 mL) water and stir to form a smooth paste. Add hot milk, vanilla and almond extract.

3. Top with marshmallows and serve immediately.

Dietitian's Message

With cinnamon, vanilla and almond extract, this is indeed the perfect cup of cocoa — and miniature marshmallows add fun. If you wish, replace sugar with an amount of artificial sweetener that has the same amount of sweetening power as 2 tsp (10 mL) sugar. Using artificial sweetener will reduce the calories to 130 and the carbohydrate content to 17 g per serving.

Exchanges Per Serving

1	Reduced-Fat Milk
1/2	Other Carbohydrate

Nutrient Analysis Per Serving

Calories	158
Protein	9 g
Fat	3 g
Saturated fat	g
Carbohydrate	24 g
Fiber	1 g
Cholesterol	10 mg
Sodium	666 mg

Hot Mulled Cider

Perfect for a Christmas party or as an après-ski drink.

4 cups	unsweetened apple juice	I L
2 tbsp	packed brown sugar	25 mL
I tsp	ground cinnamon	5 mL
½ tsp	ground nutmeg	2 mL
½ tsp	ground allspice	2 mL
10	whole cloves	10
2 to 3	cinnamon sticks	2 to 3
I	orange, sliced	I
I	lemon, sliced	I

1. In a large saucepan, over medium heat, heat apple juice, brown sugar, cinnamon, nutmeg and allspice for about 10 minutes, until simmering but not boiling.

2. Reduce heat to medium-low. Add cloves, cinnamon sticks, orange slices and lemon slices and simmer for 30 minutes or more to allow flavors to blend. Use a slotted spoon to remove the flavorings before serving.

Dietitian's Message *A hot beverage such as this is a welcome treat after a winter activity such as skiing or ice skating. To reduce the carbohydrates, replace sugar with an amount of artificial sweetener that has the same amount of sweetening power as 2 tbsp (25 mL) brown sugar. Using artificial sweetener will reduce the calories to 80 and the carbohydrate content to 20 g per serving.*

Exchanges Per Serving

1½ Fruit

Nutrient Analysis Per Serving

Calories	97
Protein	0 g
Fat	0 g
Saturated fat	0 g
Carbohydrate	24 g
Fiber	0 g
Cholesterol	0 mg
Sodium	7 mg

Frosty Chocolate Shake

- *Blender or food processor*

2 cups	vanilla ice cream	500 mL
1 cup	1% milk	250 mL
¼ cup	Chocolate Sauce (see recipe, page 159)	50 mL

1. In blender, combine ice cream, milk and Chocolate Sauce. Blend for 30 seconds, until smooth. Serve immediately.

MAKES 4 SERVINGS

A creamy chocolate shake is a perfect summer snack-time refreshment!

Exchanges Per Serving

1½ Other Carbohydrate

1 High-Fat Meat

1 Fat

Nutrient Analysis Per Serving

Calories	179
Protein	5 g
Fat	8 g
Saturated fat	5 g
Carbohydrate	23 g
Fiber	0 g
Cholesterol	32 mg
Sodium	90 mg

Chocolate soda is fun to make and absolutely delicious!

Old-Fashioned Chocolate Soda

2 tsp	unsweetened cocoa powder, sifted	10 mL
2 tsp	granulated sugar	10 mL
2 tbsp	1% milk	25 mL
½ cup	vanilla ice cream	125 mL
I	can (13 oz/355 mL) sugar-free lemon-lime soda	I

1. In a tall glass, combine cocoa and sugar. Add milk and stir until completely blended. Spoon in ice cream and slowly pour in soda. Wait until bubbles disappear, then keep adding soda slowly.

2. Serve immediately with a spoon and a straw.

Exchanges Per Serving

I ½	Other Carbohydrate
I	High-Fat Meat
I	Fat

Nutrient Analysis Per Serving

Calories	186
Protein	4 g
Fat	8 g
Saturated fat	5 g
Carbohydrate	28 g
Fiber	I g
Cholesterol	30 mg
Sodium	90 mg

Snacks and Appetizers

Black Bean Dip

When you are serving tortilla chips, this dip makes a nice change from the usual salsa and guacamole.

Tip

Be careful when using jalapeño peppers: even the fumes sting. Wash your hands promptly after handling hot peppers, and don't rub your eyes!

Variation

If you don't have a food processor, substitute refried black beans for the regular black beans and stir the ingredients together thoroughly in a mixing bowl. Be sure to read the label and select refried beans with no added fat.

- Food processor

1	can (14 oz/398 mL) black beans, drained and rinsed	1
¼ cup	lower-fat mayonnaise	50 mL
1 tbsp	freshly squeezed lime juice	15 mL
1 tsp	chili powder	5 mL
½ tsp	ground cumin	2 mL
¼ cup	diced red bell pepper	50 mL
1 tbsp	diced jalapeño pepper	15 mL
1 tbsp	chopped fresh cilantro (optional)	15 mL

1. In a food processor, blend black beans, mayonnaise, lime juice, cumin and chili powder until chunky-smooth. Add red pepper, jalapeño and cilantro, if using, and process until well mixed but still a bit chunky.

Dietitian's Message

Black beans are a good source of water-soluble fiber, which helps regulate the rise in blood sugar from a meal. Other good choices are garbanzo beans (chickpeas), navy beans, adzuki beans, white beans, kidney beans and lentils.

Exchanges Per Serving

½ Starch

Nutrient Analysis Per Serving

Calories	85
Protein	4 g
Fat	2 g
Saturated fat	0 g
Carbohydrate	13 g
Fiber	3 g
Cholesterol	0 mg
Sodium	61 mg

Hummus and Pita Chips

MAKES 8 SERVINGS
(¹/₄ cup/50 mL
hummus per serving)

- *Baking sheet*

Hummus

2	cloves garlic, minced	2
I	can (19 oz/540 mL) chickpeas, drained and rinsed	I
2 tbsp	freshly squeezed lemon juice	25 mL
2 tbsp	olive oil	25 mL
2 tbsp	plain yogurt	25 mL
¹/₂ tsp	salt	2 mL
¹/₄ tsp	hot pepper sauce	I mL
I tbsp	chopped fresh parsley	15 mL
I tsp	chopped fresh dill	5 mL
	Fresh parsley for garnish	

Pita Chips

4	6-inch (15 cm) whole wheat pitas	4
I tbsp	olive oil	15 mL
I tsp	garlic powder	5 mL

1. *Prepare the hummus:* In a food processor, purée garlic, chickpeas, lemon juice, olive oil, yogurt, salt and hot pepper sauce until smooth. Spoon into a shallow serving bowl, smooth the top and sprinkle with dill. Cover with plastic wrap and refrigerate for several hours, or overnight, to blend flavors. Garnish with parsley just before serving.

2. *Prepare the pita chips:* Preheat oven to 350°F (180°C). Cut pitas in half around the outside edge to make 8 circles. Brush with olive oil and sprinkle with garlic powder. Cut each pita into 6 wedges and arrange in a single layer on baking sheet. Bake in preheated oven for 8 to 10 minutes, or until golden. Serve with hummus.

Dietitian's Message *Chickpeas (garbanzo beans) and other legumes are a good source of soluble fiber. When served with whole wheat pita chips, the fiber content increases. Most people do not get the recommended amount of fiber in their daily food intake.*

Your guests will be impressed with your homemade, lower-fat version of this snack.

Tips

Use kitchen shears or scissors to cut pitas and tortillas.

Hummus is also great as a dip with raw vegetables.

Exchanges Per Serving

2	Starch
I	Fat

Nutrient Analysis Per Serving

Calories	211
Protein	7 g
Fat	7 g
Saturated fat	I g
Carbohydrate	33 g
Fiber	2 g
Cholesterol	0 mg
Sodium	487 mg

These chips, made from flour tortillas, are crisp and delicious. Use tortillas of different colors for even more fun!

Tips

To remove the seeds from a tomato, cut it in half crosswise, then gently scoop the seeds out.

Preparing dips a day early and chilling overnight helps to develop and blend flavors. And if you are making dips for a party, it cuts down on work the day of the festivities!

Exchanges Per Serving

I	Starch
I	Vegetable
½	Fat

Nutrient Analysis Per Serving

Calories	125
Protein	4 g
Fat	3 g
Saturated fat	0 g
Carbohydrate	22 g
Fiber	2 g
Cholesterol	0 mg
Sodium	582 mg

Salsa and Tortilla Chips

- *Preheat oven to 400°F (200°C)*
- *2 baking sheets*

Salsa

2	medium tomatoes, seeded and diced	2
I	clove garlic, minced	I
¼ cup	finely chopped onion	50 mL
2 tbsp	minced green bell pepper	25 mL
I tbsp	freshly squeezed lime juice	15 mL
I tbsp	chopped fresh cilantro (optional)	15 mL
I tsp	minced jalapeño pepper	5 mL
½ tsp	chili powder	2 mL
½ tsp	dried oregano	2 mL
½ tsp	salt	2 mL
½ tsp	freshly ground black pepper	2 mL
Dash	hot pepper sauce (optional)	Dash

Tortilla Chips

8	8-inch (20 cm) flour tortillas	8
	Olive oil spray	
I tsp	salt	5 mL
I tsp	chili powder	5 mL

1. *Prepare the salsa:* In a small non-metal bowl, combine tomatoes, garlic, onion, green pepper, lime juice, cilantro (if using), jalapeño pepper, chili powder, oregano, salt, pepper and hot pepper sauce (if using). Cover and refrigerate for at least 1 hour to blend flavors, or for up to 3 days. Makes 1 cup (250 mL).

2. *Prepare the tortilla chips:* Lightly spray both sides of tortillas with olive oil spray. Cut each tortilla into 8 wedges. Arrange in a single layer on baking sheets; bake for 5 minutes, until crisp and lightly browned. Serve with salsa.

> ### Dietitian's Message
> *This fresh and lively salsa can be used with all of your favorite Mexican dishes and 2 tbsp (25 mL) provides only 10 calories and 2 grams of carbohydrate. The homemade chips are low in fat and a lot more satisfying than store-bought fried tortilla chips.*

Guacamole Nachos

You can adjust the heat to your liking by adding more or less hot pepper sauce.

Tip

For the best flavor and ease in preparation, be sure to use ripe avocados. You'll know they're ripe if the flesh yields when gently squeezed. Hard avocados can be ripened by burying them in flour for 1 to 2 days.

- Preheat oven to 350°F (180°C)
- Rimmed baking sheets

2	green onions, chopped	2
I	large tomato, diced	I
I	avocado, diced	I
I	clove garlic, minced	I
I tbsp	chopped fresh cilantro (optional)	15 mL
I tbsp	freshly squeezed lemon juice	15 mL
¼ tsp	hot pepper sauce	I mL
6	8-inch (20 cm) flour tortillas	6
	Olive oil spray	
I cup	shredded part-skim mozzarella cheese, divided	250 mL

I. In a small bowl, combine green onions, tomato, avocado, garlic, cilantro (if using), lemon juice and hot pepper sauce.

2. Lightly spray both sides of tortillas with olive oil spray and cut each into 6 wedges. Arrange in a single layer on baking sheets and bake in preheated oven for 5 minutes, until crisp and lightly browned. Sprinkle ½ cup (125 mL) of the mozzarella evenly over the chips; bake for 3 minutes, until cheese is melted.

3. Spoon 1 tbsp (15 mL) of the guacamole mixture onto each chip and sprinkle the remaining ½ cup (125 mL) mozzarella evenly over the guacamole. Return to the oven and continue baking for 5 minutes, until nachos are heated through and cheese is melted.

Exchanges Per Serving

I	Starch
I	Vegetable
I	High-Fat Meat
½	Fat

Nutrient Analysis Per Serving

Calories	229
Protein	9 g
Fat	11 g
Saturated fat	3 g
Carbohydrate	25 g
Fiber	2 g
Cholesterol	10 mg
Sodium	260 mg

Dietitian's Message *The avocado in this guacamole adds to the fat content; however, avocados are especially high in the healthier monounsaturated fats. They also contain calcium, protein and healthy doses of vitamins A, B and C.*

Quick Quesadillas

2	8-inch (20 cm) flour tortillas	2
2 tbsp	salsa (store-bought or see recipe, page 58)	25 mL
¼ cup	shredded part-skim mozzarella or Cheddar cheese	50 mL
1 tbsp	chopped green onion	15 mL
¼ cup	1% cottage cheese	50 mL

1. Place one tortilla on a microwave-safe plate. Spread with salsa and sprinkle with mozzarella and green onion. Spoon on cottage cheese and top with the second tortilla.

2. Microwave, uncovered, on Medium-High (70%) for 40 seconds to 1 minute, or until mozzarella is melted. Cut into quarters and serve.

Dietitian's Message *This recipe is easy for an older child or teen to put together. It's delicious, quick and satisfying. Eaten as an after-school snack, it provides enough protein and carbohydrate to keep a hungry teen going until dinnertime.*

Say "¡Sí!" to a little spicy variety for lunch or snacks.

Tip
Microwave ovens vary in power, so the cooking time will vary as well. Always start with the shortest time.

Variation
For a great addition to a Mexican BBQ, these quesadillas can be cooked on the grill. Brush the grill with vegetable oil and then grill quesadillas, uncovered, over medium heat for 2 to 3 minutes per side, turning once, until the cheese melts and the tortilla is crispy. Cut into wedges and serve as an appetizer.

Exchanges Per Serving

1½ Starch

1½ Medium-Fat Meat

Nutrient Analysis Per Serving

Calories	225
Protein	15 g
Fat	8 g
Saturated fat	4 g
Carbohydrate	22 g
Fiber	2 g
Cholesterol	21 mg
Sodium	461 mg

Potato Skins

These nutritious and satisfying potato skins are a great snack to serve your kids and their friends while they're watching the big game on TV.

Variation

Italian Potato Skins: Substitute equal amounts of chopped green bell peppers for the corn, garbanzo beans (chickpeas) for the black beans, and spaghetti or marinara sauce for the salsa.

- Preheat oven to 400°F (200°C)
- Baking sheet

6	small baking potatoes, scrubbed	6
1 tsp	chili powder	5 mL
1 cup	salsa (store-bought or see recipe, page 58)	250 mL
¾ cup	drained, rinsed canned black beans	175 mL
½ cup	frozen corn kernels, thawed	125 mL
1½ cup	shredded part-skim mozzarella or Cheddar cheese	375 mL
½ cup	lower-fat sour cream (optional)	125 mL

1. Pierce the potatoes with a sharp knife and bake directly on the oven rack in preheated oven until tender, about 45 minutes. Let cool. Meanwhile, preheat the broiler and position the oven rack 6 inches (15 cm) from the element.

2. Cut potatoes lengthwise. Using a small spoon, scoop out all but ¼ inch (0.5 cm) of the potato, being careful not to break the skin. Save the potato pulp for another use. Cut each shell into 4 wedges and arrange in a single layer on baking sheet. Lightly spray potatoes with vegetable spray and sprinkle with chili powder. Broil for 5 minutes.

Exchanges Per Serving

½ Starch
2 Lean Meat
½ Fat

Nutrient Analysis Per Serving

Calories	183
Protein	15 g
Fat	8 g
Saturated fat	5 g
Carbohydrate	13 g
Fiber	3 g
Cholesterol	29 mg
Sodium	309 mg

3. In a medium bowl, combine salsa, black beans and corn. Spoon onto potato skins, dividing mixture evenly, and sprinkle with mozzarella. Return to the oven and broil for 3 to 4 minutes, or until cheese melts.

4. Serve with sour cream, if using.

Dietitian's Message *These potato skins can be enjoyed for dinner as a side dish or as an evening party snack. Eaten before bed, the combination of protein and carbohydrate, in addition to the water-soluble fiber in the black beans, makes this recipe particularly beneficial for maintaining blood sugar overnight, with less chance of it dropping too low. A milder salsa might decrease the chances of heartburn though!*

Mini Pizzas

Quick and easy to prepare, these mini pizzas make a great lunch, after-school snack or even breakfast!

Variation

Experiment with your favorite toppings. Here are some ideas: Swiss cheese and bacon bits, sliced wieners and Cheddar, ham and pineapple, pepperoni and mushrooms.

- Broiler or toaster oven
- Baking sheet

½ cup	shredded part-skim mozzarella cheese	125 mL
2 tbsp	grated Parmesan cheese	25 mL
½ tsp	dried Italian seasoning	2 mL
2	English muffins	2
¼ cup	pizza or spaghetti sauce	50 mL
½ tsp	garlic powder	2 mL
¼ cup	diced lean ham	50 mL

1. Preheat the broiler with the oven rack 5 to 6 inches (13 to 15 cm) from the element (or use a toaster oven.)
2. In a small bowl, mix mozzarella, Parmesan and Italian seasoning.
3. Cut English muffins in half, place on baking sheet, and toast cut side up under the broiler until golden.
4. Spread each muffin with 1 tbsp (15 mL) pizza sauce, sprinkle with garlic powder and top with ¼ of the cheese mixture and 1 tbsp (15 mL) ham.
5. Broil for 3 to 4 minutes, until the cheese melts.

Exchanges Per Serving

1	Starch
2	Medium-Fat Meat

Nutrient Analysis Per Serving

Calories	213
Protein	16 g
Fat	9 g
Saturated fat	5 g
Carbohydrate	17 g
Fiber	0 g
Cholesterol	31 mg
Sodium	619 mg

Caesar Salad (page 71) ▶
Overleaf: Frosty Strawberry Shake (page 47)

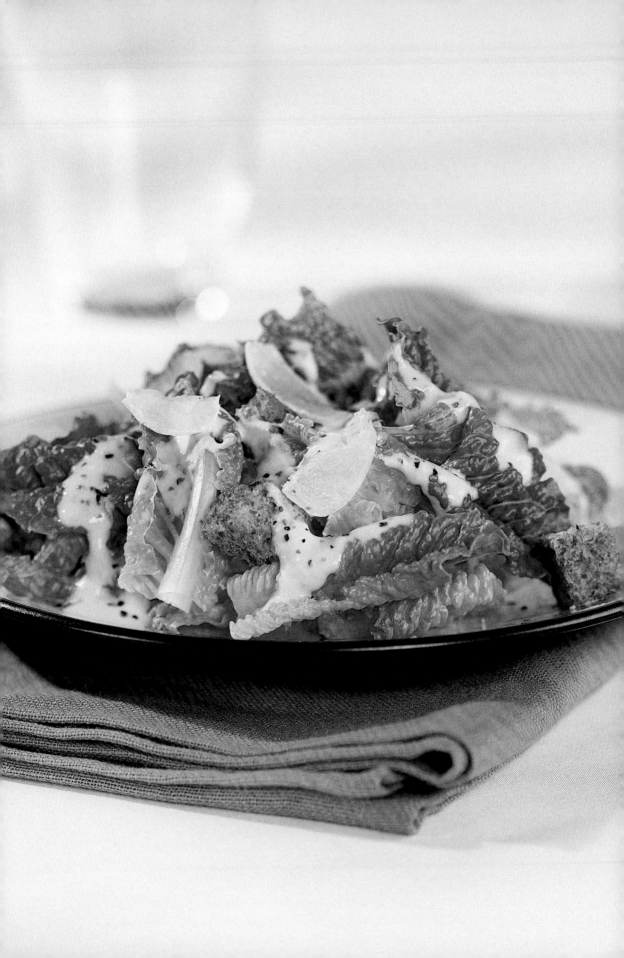

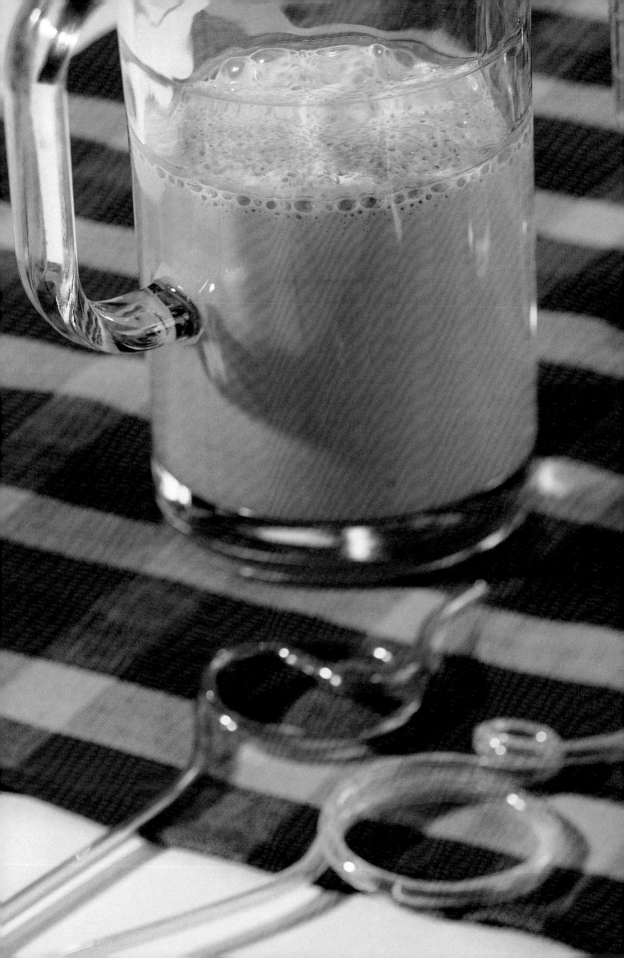

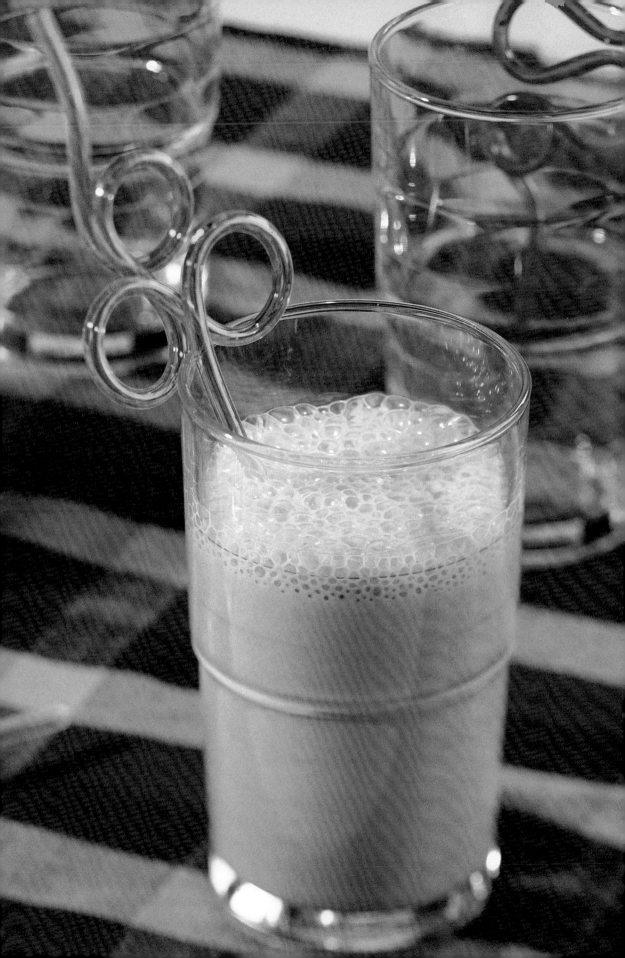

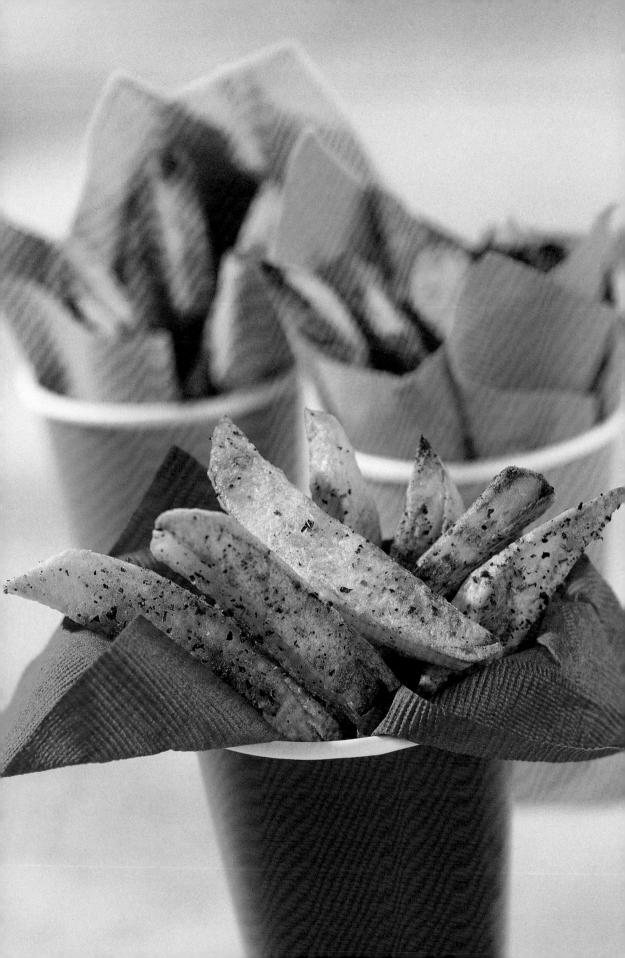

Fast and Spicy Pizza Bagels

3	bagels (each 3 oz/90 g), split	3
1/4 cup	pizza or spaghetti sauce	50 mL
6	green bell pepper rings	6
6	red bell pepper rings	6
6	red onion rings (or to taste)	6
1 1/4 cup	shredded jalapeño-flavored Monterey Jack cheese	300 mL

1. Cut each bagel in half and spread each half lightly with pizza sauce. Top each with 1 green pepper ring, 1 red pepper ring and 1 onion ring. Sprinkle with Monterey Jack.

2. On a microwave-safe plate covered with paper towels, microwave 3 bagel halves at a time, uncovered, on High for 1 to 2 minutes, or until cheese is melted and bagel is hot.

Dietitian's Message *These pizzas are great for a quick snack. For a full meal, add a serving of salad with vinaigrette dressing.*

This is a great after-school snack for hungry teens because it is fast and easy to make in the microwave.

Variation

These pizza bagels can be as varied as much as your imagination allows! Add mushrooms, tomatoes, pineapple and ham or feta and spinach. If jalapeño-flavored Monterey Jack is too spicy for your taste, substitute your favorite cheese.

Exchanges Per Serving

1 1/2 Starch
1 Vegetable
1/2 Medium-Fat Meat
1/2 Fat

Nutrient Analysis Per Serving

Calories	234
Protein	11 g
Fat	8 g
Saturated fat	5 g
Carbohydrate	29 g
Fiber	2 g
Cholesterol	21 mg
Sodium	396 mg

◀ Oven French Fries (page 78)

Buffalo Wings

Buffalo wings are normally deep-fried; this version is broiled, helping to keep the fats lower! If these wings are too hot for you, decrease the amount of hot pepper sauce.

Tip

When broiling food, keep the oven door slightly ajar and be very cautious. Never let your children broil fatty food without constant adult supervision.

- Broiler
- Broiler pan, sprayed with vegetable spray

12	chicken wings	12
2 tbsp	soft margarine	25 mL
2 tbsp	hot pepper sauce	25 mL
1 tsp	paprika	5 mL
½ tsp	salt	2 mL
¼ tsp	freshly ground black pepper	1 mL
	Lower-fat or no-fat ranch or blue cheese salad dressing	

1. Rinse the chicken wings and pat dry with paper towels. Cut each at the joints into 3 pieces and discard the wing tips, leaving 24 pieces. Place in a shallow non-metal bowl.

2. In a small microwave-safe bowl, microwave margarine on High for 20 to 30 seconds, until melted. Stir in hot pepper sauce and paprika.

3. Pour sauce over the wings. Stir to coat, cover and refrigerate for at least 30 minutes or for up to 8 hours.

4. Preheat the broiler with the broiler pan 8 inches (20 cm) from the element. Arrange chicken pieces on the rack of the broiler pan. Sprinkle with salt and pepper and brush with any leftover sauce.

5. Broil for 10 to 15 minutes, until light brown. Turn the pieces, and broil for about 10 minutes longer, until juices run clear when chicken is pierced with a fork and skin is crisp.

6. Serve with ranch or blue cheese salad dressing as a dipping sauce.

Exchanges Per Serving

2	High-Fat Meat

Nutrient Analysis Per Serving

Calories	253
Protein	18 g
Fat	20 g
Saturated fat	5 g
Carbohydrate	0 g
Fiber	0 g
Cholesterol	76 mg
Sodium	413 mg

Dietitian's Message *Wow, no carbs! For those who count carbohydrates, these wings can be eaten as a bonus snack. Of course, they do have calories and fat, so watch the portion size and the dips you choose.*

Spicy Popcorn

- *Hot-air popper*

½ cup	popcorn kernels	125 mL
2 tsp	chili powder	10 mL
1 tsp	garlic powder	5 mL
1 tsp	salt	5 mL
1 tbsp	vegetable oil	15 mL

1. Pop popcorn kernels in hot-air popper and pour into a large serving bowl. (You should have about 16 cups/4 L.)

2. While the popcorn is popping, in a small bowl, stir together chili powder, garlic powder and salt.

3. Sprinkle vegetable oil onto the hot popped corn and toss gently. Add the spice mixture and toss again until evenly coated.

ALTERNATIVE METHOD

1. If you don't have a hot-air popper, you can make popcorn on the stove using a very large saucepan with a heavy bottom and a tight-fitting lid. Heat 1 tbsp (15 mL) vegetable oil over medium-high heat. Add one popcorn kernel and wait for it to pop. Immediately add the remaining kernels, cover and lower heat to medium-low. Shaking occasionally, allow corn to pop. Listen carefully, and when popping has almost stopped, remove from heat and pour popcorn into a bowl, discarding any unpopped kernels. Be aware that your popcorn will have less volume, so serving sizes will be smaller.

Here's a fun way to jazz up your popcorn.

Tip

An easy way to mix the popcorn with the spices is to place them in a large paper bag and shake gently.

Exchanges Per Serving

1½ Starch

Nutrient Analysis Per Serving

Calories	137
Protein	4 g
Fat	3 g
Saturated fat	0 g
Carbohydrate	26 g
Fiber	5 g
Cholesterol	0 mg
Sodium	287 mg

Holiday Cut-outs

Use this recipe to make festive snacks for Christmas (or spooky treats for Halloween).

Variation

For Halloween, cut bread into ghost shapes and substitute 12 black olives for the peppers. Cut pitted olives into 3 slices each, and use the center slice for an open mouth and the 2 end slices for eyes.

- Preheat broiler
- Baking sheet

12	thin slices white bread	12
3 tbsp	lower-fat mayonnaise	45 mL
1 tsp	dried dillweed	5 mL
1 tsp	garlic powder	5 mL
1 cup	shredded part-skim mozzarella cheese	250 mL
1/2 cup	diced red and green bell peppers	125 mL

1. With a sharp knife or using a large cookie cutter, cut bread into shapes such as Christmas trees, hearts, stars, etc. You should use about $2/3$ of a slice of bread for each cut-out and discard the rest.

2. In a small bowl, combine mayonnaise, dill and garlic powder.

3. Position the oven rack 6 inches (15 cm) from the element. Arrange shapes on baking sheet and broil for 1 to 2 minutes, or until lightly browned.

4. Flip toasted shapes and spread with mayonnaise mixture. Sprinkle with mozzarella and peppers. Broil for another 1 to 2 minutes, or until cheese melts. Serve warm.

Dietitian's Message

This fun snack can be made to suit any special time of the year, be it Halloween, Christmas, Valentine's Day or a birthday. Be creative! Children can help prepare these cut-out treats — and when they've helped make something, they're more likely to taste and eat it. For a little more fiber, use whole wheat bread.

Exchanges Per Serving

1	Starch
1	Vegetable
1	Fat

Nutrient Analysis Per Serving

Calories	170
Protein	8 g
Fat	6 g
Saturated fat	2 g
Carbohydrate	20 g
Fiber	1 g
Cholesterol	12 mg
Sodium	320 mg

Salads and
Side Dishes

Carrot Salad

Enjoy the zippy taste of the dressing over the grated carrots and parsley. This colorful salad is great for picnics and potlucks because it can be made early in the day and chilled until serving time.

Tip

Most dressings can be prepared in advance and refrigerated for up to 3 days. Small glass jars are great containers. Put dressing ingredients in a jar with a tight-fitting lid, refrigerate and shake well just before using.

Variation

Add ½ cup (125 mL) raisins with the carrots and parsley and serve on a bed of lettuce.

| 2 cups | grated carrots | 500 mL |
| 2 tbsp | chopped fresh parsley | 25 mL |

Dressing

1 tbsp	freshly squeezed lemon juice	15 mL
1 tbsp	white wine vinegar	15 mL
1 tbsp	vegetable oil	15 mL
1 tsp	granulated sugar	5 mL
½ tsp	Dijon mustard	2 mL
¼ tsp	salt	1 mL
¼ tsp	freshly ground black pepper	1 mL

1. In a medium glass bowl, combine carrots and parsley.
2. *Prepare the dressing:* In a small bowl, whisk together lemon juice, vinegar, oil, sugar, mustard, salt and pepper.
3. Pour dressing over carrots and parsley and toss to coat. Cover and refrigerate for at least 1 hour or for up to 8 hours.

Dietitian's Message *One serving of this salad will meet your requirement of vitamin A for the day.*

Exchanges Per Serving

| 1 | Vegetable |
| ½ | Fat |

Nutrient Analysis Per Serving

Calories	60
Protein	1 g
Fat	4 g
Saturated fat	0 g
Carbohydrate	7 g
Fiber	1 g
Cholesterol	0 mg
Sodium	172 mg

Caesar Salad

Caesar Dressing

¾ cup	1% cottage cheese	175 mL
2	cloves garlic, minced	2
2 tbsp	freshly squeezed lemon juice	25 mL
1½ tsp	Dijon mustard	7 mL
1 tsp	anchovy paste	5 mL
1 tsp	Worcestershire sauce	5 mL
½ tsp	salt	2 mL
½ tsp	freshly ground black pepper	2 mL
2 tsp	olive oil	10 mL
1 tbsp	lower-fat sour cream	15 mL
¼ cup	freshly grated Parmesan cheese	50 mL

Quick Croutons

2	slices whole wheat bread	2
2 tsp	olive oil	10 mL
½ tsp	garlic powder	2 mL
½ tsp	dried Italian seasoning	2 mL

Salad

8 cups	torn romaine lettuce (about 2 medium heads)	2 L
¼ cup	freshly grated Parmesan cheese	50 mL

1. *Prepare the dressing:* In a food processor or blender, purée cottage cheese until smooth. Blend in garlic, lemon juice, mustard, anchovy paste, salt and pepper. Add olive oil and blend until thick and smooth. Add sour cream and Parmesan and blend just until mixed. Cover and refrigerate for at least 1 hour or for up to 1 day.

2. *Prepare the croutons:* Cut bread into cubes. In a glass pie plate, toss bread cubes with olive oil, garlic powder and Italian seasoning. Microwave, covered with a paper towel, on High, stopping twice to stir, for 3 to 4 minutes, or until crisp.

3. *Prepare the salad:* Place lettuce in a large salad bowl, pour in dressing and toss. Sprinkle with Parmesan and croutons, toss lightly and serve immediately.

Everybody's favorite salad, with a lower-fat creamy dressing!

Tips

Caesar salad must be eaten immediately after tossing or it goes limp. Prepare the lettuce ahead and keep it crisp in a plastic bag with a paper towel inside. Make the dressing ahead and keep it in the refrigerator until ready to toss with the salad.

The croutons can also be made in advance and stored at room temperature in an airtight container for up to 1 week.

Exchanges Per Serving

1	Vegetable
1	Lean Meat
½	Fat

Nutrient Analysis Per Serving

Calories	98
Protein	7 g
Fat	5 g
Saturated fat	2 g
Carbohydrate	7 g
Fiber	2 g
Cholesterol	6 mg
Sodium	430 mg

Pasta Salad on a Stick

Why is it that putting food on a stick improves the flavor? This is a fun salad to make and to serve.

- *Twelve 10-inch (25 cm) skewers*

7 oz	fresh spinach tortellini	200 g
24	cherry tomatoes	24
12	pitted jumbo black olives	12
2	red or green bell peppers, cut into 1-inch (2.5 cm) cubes	2
1/4 cup	lower-fat Italian dressing	50 mL
3 oz	part-skim mozzarella cheese, cut into 1/2-inch (1 cm) cubes (about 2/3 cup/150 mL)	90 g
4 oz	turkey salami, thinly sliced	125 g

1. In a medium saucepan, cook tortellini in boiling salted water according to package directions. Drain and rinse with cold water to stop cooking.

2. Place tortellini, tomatoes, olives and peppers in a shallow glass dish. Drizzle with Italian dressing and marinate at room temperature for 30 minutes. Add mozzarella and salami. Gently toss to coat with dressing.

3. Cut turkey salami slices in half and then fold in half.

4. Alternately thread tortellini, tomatoes, peppers, cheese cubes and folded salami slices on skewers. Top each skewer with an olive. Serve immediately or refrigerate for up to 2 hours, until ready to serve.

Exchanges Per Serving

1 1/2 Starch

1 Vegetable

1 Medium-Fat Meat

Nutrient Analysis Per Serving

Calories	243
Protein	12 g
Fat	7 g
Saturated fat	3 g
Carbohydrate	34 g
Fiber	5 g
Cholesterol	25 mg
Sodium	555 mg

Taco Salad

10 oz	lean ground turkey	300 g
²⁄₃ cup	salsa, divided (store-bought, or see recipe, page 58)	150 mL
1 tbsp	chili powder	15 mL
8	romaine lettuce leaves, coarsely chopped	8
4 oz	plain tortilla chips (about 5 cups/1.25 L)	125 g
4	green onions, sliced	4
2	medium tomatoes, diced	2
½ cup	cooked black beans, drained and rinsed (if using canned)	125 mL
½ cup	shredded lower-fat Cheddar cheese	125 mL
⅓ cup	lower-fat sour cream	75 mL

The great taste of tacos is easy to reproduce in a refreshing salad.

Tip

As a general rule, salad greens should be torn and not cut with a knife. Cutting bruises the lettuce and causes it to go brown. In recipes that call for chopped lettuce (such as this one) use a stainless steel knife and serve as soon as possible to minimize the browning.

1. In a medium nonstick skillet, over medium-high heat, brown ground turkey, stirring often and breaking up until crumbly, for 5 to 6 minutes, or until no longer pink. Reduce heat to low, stir in ½ cup (125 mL) of the salsa and chili powder and simmer for 10 minutes.

2. Divide lettuce among 4 dinner plates. Surround with tortilla chips. Spoon hot turkey mixture onto lettuce and top with green onions, tomatoes, beans, Cheddar, sour cream and the remaining ¼ cup (50 mL) salsa.

Dietitian's Message *For less fat in this Taco Salad, substitute homemade tortilla chips (see recipe, page 58).*

Exchanges Per Serving

1½	Starch
1	Vegetable
2½	Lean Meat
2	Fat

Nutrient Analysis Per Serving

Calories	374
Protein	23 g
Fat	18 g
Saturated fat	5 g
Carbohydrate	32 g
Fiber	6 g
Cholesterol	70 mg
Sodium	436 mg

Chicken Salad Nests

Prepare the chicken salad an hour before serving, but assemble the salad on the nest just before serving so that the noodles will be crisp.

Tip

When choosing fruit and vegetables for your salads, always select the freshest available. They will taste the best and have the most nutrients.

Variation

Substitute 2 cans (each 6 oz /170 g) drained, water-packed chunky light or white tuna for the chicken.

2½ cups	cooked diced chicken breasts (about 8 oz/250 g)	625 mL
1 cup	halved red or green seedless grapes	250 mL
½ cup	drained pineapple tidbits	125 mL
¼ cup	diced celery	50 mL
2 tbsp	plain yogurt	25 mL
2 tbsp	lower-fat mayonnaise	25 mL
½ tsp	salt	2 mL
1½ cups	crisp chow mein noodles	375 mL
½ cup	grated carrots	125 mL
2 tbsp	chopped fresh chives or parsley	25 mL

1. In a medium bowl, mix chicken, grapes, pineapple and celery.

2. In a small bowl, combine yogurt, mayonnaise and salt. Pour over chicken mixture and toss lightly. Cover and refrigerate for 1 hour.

3. Just before serving, combine noodles and carrots. Divide evenly among 4 serving plates. Mound chicken mixture in the middle of each "nest" and sprinkle with chives.

Dietitian's Message *Pineapple packed in syrup has more sugar than pineapple packed in its own juice. For less carbohydrate, use canned fruit packed in its own juice or in pear juice.*

Exchanges Per Serving

1	Starch
½	Fruit
2½	Lean Meat

Nutrient Analysis Per Serving

Calories	245
Protein	21 g
Fat	9 g
Saturated fat	1 g
Carbohydrate	22 g
Fiber	2 g
Cholesterol	53 mg
Sodium	443 mg

Chicken Fajita Salad

- 6 ovenproof bowls, 2 baking sheets and broiler pan, lined with foil

2	cloves garlic, minced	2
2 tsp	vegetable oil	10 mL
2 tbsp	freshly squeezed lime juice	25 mL
1 tbsp	granulated sugar	15 mL
2 tsp	chili powder	10 mL
4	skinless boneless chicken breasts (about 1 lb/500 g)	4
	Vegetable spray	
6	8-inch (20 cm) flour tortillas	6
4 cups	shredded lettuce	1 L
12	pitted black olives, sliced (optional)	12
3	green onions, sliced	3
2	medium tomatoes, diced	2
1	avocado, diced	1
	Salsa (store-bought or see recipe, page 58)	
	Lower-fat sour cream (optional)	

Try making this salad for a birthday party. It looks special and tastes delicious. Teens might prefer to eat this as a wrap. Omit Step 2 and use the plain tortillas to wrap the prepared ingredients.

Tip

If you don't have ovenproof bowls you can use, scrunch 6 pieces of aluminum foil into large balls (about 4 inches/10 cm in diameter) and use them instead.

1. In a shallow dish, combine garlic, oil, lime juice, sugar and chili powder. Add chicken and turn to coat both sides. Cover and refrigerate for 1 to 2 hours. Meanwhile, preheat oven to 400°F (200°C).

2. Invert ovenproof bowls on cookie sheets and spray with vegetable spray. Place one tortilla over each bowl (tortillas will mold to bowls while baking). Spray with vegetable spray. Bake in preheated oven for 6 to 7 minutes, or until crisp and golden. Remove tortillas from bowls and cool. Preheat broiler with the rack 6 inches (15 cm) from the element.

3. Place marinated chicken on broiler pan, discarding marinade. Broil for 8 minutes. Turn and broil the other side for 7 to 8 minutes, or until chicken reaches an internal temperature of 170°F (75°C) and is no longer pink inside. Cut into strips.

4. Divide lettuce evenly among tortilla shells. Top with chicken, olives (if using), green onions, tomatoes and avocado. Serve with salsa and sour cream, if using.

Exchanges Per Serving

1½ Starch

2½ Meat and Meat Substitute

1½ Fat

Nutrient Analysis Per Serving

Calories	303
Protein	22 g
Fat	12 g
Saturated fat	2 g
Carbohydrate	29 g
Fiber	3 g
Cholesterol	44 mg
Sodium	250 mg

Ham Fried Rice

This is a very quick dish when you need to prepare a meal in a hurry. Cook the rice up to 1 day in advance or use leftover rice from a previous meal. Serve as part of a Chinese dinner, or add more ham and peas for a complete one-pot meal.

Tip

Leftover meat and vegetables from last night's meal make easy additions to fried rice.

Variation

Substitute an equal amount of cooked chicken, shrimp or tofu for the ham.

2 tsp	vegetable oil, divided	10 mL
3	large eggs	3
½ cup	grated carrots	125 mL
½ cup	sliced mushrooms	125 mL
¼ cup	chopped celery	50 mL
½ cup	diced lean cooked ham (about 2 oz/60 g)	125 mL
¼ cup	sliced green onions	50 mL
3 cups	cooked long-grain rice (1 cup/250 mL raw)	750 mL
½ cup	frozen peas	125 mL
3 tbsp	sodium-reduced soy sauce	45 mL

1. In a large nonstick skillet or wok, heat 1 tsp (5 mL) of the oil over medium heat.

2. In a small bowl, beat eggs with a fork. Pour into skillet and cook (like a thin omelet) until set. Remove from skillet, cut into thin strips and set aside.

3. Heat the remaining 1 tsp (5 mL) oil and sauté carrots, mushrooms and celery for 5 minutes, until mushrooms are soft. Stir in ham and green onions and cook for 1 minute more, just until onions soften slightly.

4. Add rice and peas. Sprinkle with soy sauce and toss gently. Stir in scrambled eggs. Reduce heat to medium-low. Cover and cook for 5 minutes, until heated through.

Dietitian's Message *Substitute whatever vegetables you have on hand for the ones in the recipe. Keep in mind, though, that some vegetables add carbohydrate and some add little carbohydrate.*

Exchanges Per Serving

1½ Starch

1   Lean Meat

Nutrient Analysis Per Serving

Calories	202
Protein	11 g
Fat	6 g
Saturated fat	1 g
Carbohydrate	26 g
Fiber	2 g
Cholesterol	119 mg
Sodium	604 mg

Smashed Potatoes

1 ½ lbs	red-skinned potatoes (about 5 medium)	750 g
1 tsp	chicken stock powder	5 mL
2	green onions, chopped	2
½ cup	plain yogurt	125 mL
2 tbsp	butter	25 mL
1 tsp	salt	5 mL
½ tsp	freshly ground black pepper	2 mL
2 tbsp	chopped fresh parsley	25 mL

By cooking the potatoes with their skins on, you keep all of the fiber and nutrients while adding texture and flavor.

Tip

To turn this into a vegetarian recipe, use vegetable stock powder instead of chicken stock powder.

1. Scrub potatoes well and cut out any black spots. Cut into 1- to 1½-inch (2.5 to 4 cm) cubes. Place in a large saucepan with just enough water to cover, add stock powder and bring to a boil. Reduce heat to low and simmer, covered, for 20 to 25 minutes, or until tender. Drain well.

2. In the same saucepan, mash the potatoes. Add green onions, yogurt, butter, salt and pepper. Beat with a wooden spoon until light and fluffy. Stir in fresh parsley and serve.

Dietitian's Message

A potato's ability to raise blood sugar depends on the type of potato and how it is prepared. Mashing potatoes makes them more easily digestible, and they raise blood sugar more quickly. Leaving the peel on the potatoes and consuming fat, vegetables and milk at the same meal will help to slow and reduce the blood sugar rise.

Exchanges Per Serving

2	Starch
1	Fat

Nutrient Analysis Per Serving

Calories	198
Protein	6 g
Fat	6 g
Saturated fat	4 g
Carbohydrate	31 g
Fiber	3 g
Cholesterol	16 mg
Sodium	989 mg

The taste and crispiness of french fries without the fat!

Tip

Soaking potatoes in cold water removes some starch, which results in crispier fries.

Variation

Parmesan Potatoes:
Cut potatoes into thinner (¼-inch/0.5 cm) strips. Proceed as above, but turn after 15 minutes, sprinkle lightly with 2 tbsp (25 mL) freshly grated Parmesan cheese and continue baking for 15 minutes, until crisp and golden.

Oven French Fries

- *Preheat oven to 450°F (230°C)*
- *Baking sheet, sprayed with vegetable spray*

2 lbs	baking potatoes, peeled (about 5 large)	I kg
4 tsp	olive oil	20 mL
	Salt or seasoning salt	

1. Cut potatoes lengthwise into ½-inch (1 cm) strips. Soak in a large bowl of cold water for at least 15 minutes. (Or let them soak, refrigerated, until ready to use. Make sure they are completely immersed so they won't go brown.) Drain and pat dry with paper towels.

2. Toss potatoes with olive oil and arrange in a single layer on prepared baking sheet. Bake in preheated oven for 20 minutes. Turn and continue baking for 15 minutes, until crisp and golden. Sprinkle with salt and serve.

Dietitian's Message *These fries taste scrumptious and have an impressively low fat content compared to regular french fries, saving many calories and helping decrease overall fat intake for the day.*

Exchanges Per Serving

2	Starch
½	Fat

Nutrient Analysis Per Serving

Calories	175
Protein	4 g
Fat	4 g
Saturated fat	I g
Carbohydrate	33 g
Fiber	3 g
Cholesterol	0 mg
Sodium	120 mg

Stuffed Baked Potatoes

- Preheat oven to 400°F (200°C)
- 13- by 9-inch (3 L) baking dish

4	medium baking potatoes (about 1⅓ lbs/670 g)	4
¼ cup	1% cottage cheese	50 mL
2 tbsp	minced chives or green onions	25 mL
2 tbsp	plain yogurt	25 mL
½ tsp	salt	2 mL
¼ tsp	freshly ground black pepper	1 mL
¼ cup	shredded part-skim mozzarella or Cheddar cheese	50 mL

1. Scrub potatoes well. Pierce each with a large fork and bake for 50 to 60 minutes, or until tender. Let cool. Reduce oven temperature to 350°F (180°C).

2. Cut potatoes in half lengthwise. Using a small spoon, scoop out all but ¼ inch (0.5 cm) of the potato, being careful not to break the skin. Place potato shells in baking dish.

3. In a medium bowl, mash potato pulp with a fork or potato masher. Add cottage cheese, chives, yogurt, salt and pepper. Mix well, then spoon back into the potato shells. Sprinkle evenly with mozzarella.

4. Return potatoes to the oven and bake for 15 minutes, or until cheese is melted and potato is heated through.

Dietitian's Message *The cottage cheese, yogurt, and mozzarella or Cheddar lower the glycemic response of the baked potato, helping to keep blood sugar level and averting a sharp rise after eating.*

MAKES 4 SERVINGS

Kids like to make (and eat) these potatoes that turn an ordinary dinner into a fancy one!

Tip

You can also heat these potatoes on the barbecue. Instead of returning them to the oven for the final stage of baking, place them on a sheet of aluminum foil and grill for 15 minutes while barbecuing the main course.

Exchanges Per Serving

1½ Starch
½ Very Lean Meat

Nutrient Analysis Per Serving

Calories	145
Protein	7 g
Fat	2 g
Saturated fat	1 g
Carbohydrate	26 g
Fiber	2 g
Cholesterol	5 mg
Sodium	380 mg

Prepare this casserole early in the day and serve it at suppertime. It goes well with a roast beef, ham or turkey dinner.

Tip

To make ahead, prepare recipe early in the day, cover and refrigerate for up to 8 hours. Uncover before baking and increase the baking time by 10 minutes.

Variation

Substitute Yukon gold potatoes. They have a rich, buttery flavor and are great for mashing.

Exchanges Per Serving

1½ Starch
1 Lean Meat
½ Fat

Nutrient Analysis Per Serving

Calories	181
Protein	11 g
Fat	6 g
Saturated fat	2 g
Carbohydrate	22 g
Fiber	2 g
Cholesterol	79 mg
Sodium	393 mg

Mashed Potato Casserole

- *8-cup (2 L) casserole dish, sprayed with vegetable spray*

6	medium baking potatoes, peeled (about 2 lbs/1 kg)	6
1 tbsp	soft margarine	15 mL
2	large eggs	2
½ cup	1% cottage cheese	125 mL
¾ cup	shredded lower-fat Cheddar cheese	175 mL
¼ cup	lower-fat sour cream	50 mL
½ tsp	salt	2 mL
½ tsp	freshly ground black pepper	2 mL
¼ tsp	ground nutmeg	1 mL

1. Cut potatoes into quarters and place in a medium saucepan. Add just enough water to cover and 1 tsp (5 mL) salt. Bring to a boil, then reduce heat to medium-low. Cover and simmer for 25 minutes, until tender. Drain well. Preheat oven to 400°F (200°C).

2. Mash potatoes well with a potato masher and mix in margarine.

3. In a food processor or blender, purée eggs and cottage cheese. Stir into mashed potatoes. Add Cheddar, sour cream, salt, pepper and nutmeg and mix well.

4. Spoon potato mixture into prepared casserole dish. Bake in preheated oven, uncovered, for 25 minutes, until piping hot and slightly browned.

Dietitian's Message *Using lower-fat Cheddar cheese, lower-fat sour cream and 1% cottage cheese halves the fat in this dish, and the taste is really no different.*

Potato Pancakes

4	medium baking potatoes, peeled (about 1 1/2 lbs/750 g)	4
1/2 cup	grated carrots	125 mL
2 tbsp	grated onion	25 mL
1/3 cup	all-purpose flour	75 mL
1 tsp	salt	5 mL
1/2 tsp	baking powder	2 mL
2	large eggs	2
1/3 cup	1% milk	75 mL
2 tbsp	vegetable oil, divided	25 mL
1/2 cup	unsweetened applesauce	125 mL
1/2 cup	lower-fat sour cream	125 mL

1. Cut potatoes into quarters and place in a medium saucepan. Add just enough water to cover and 1 tsp (5 mL) salt. Bring to a boil, then reduce heat to medium-low. Cover and simmer for 20 minutes, until just tender. Drain and let cool.

2. In a large bowl, grate the cooled potatoes and combine with carrots and onion.

3. In a small bowl, stir together flour, salt and baking powder. Add to potatoes and toss with a fork to mix.

4. In the same small bowl, beat eggs and milk. Stir into potato mixture until well blended.

5. In a large nonstick skillet or on a griddle, heat 1 tbsp (15 mL) of the oil over medium heat. Using 1/2 the batter, scoop 4 mounds into the hot skillet. Using a spatula, flatten to 1/2 inch (1 cm). Fry for 6 to 8 minutes per side, turning only once, until deep golden.

6. Transfer to a paper towel–lined plate and keep warm. Add the remaining 1 tbsp (15 mL) oil to the skillet and repeat with the remaining batter.

7. Serve topped with applesauce and sour cream.

Dietitian's Message *For a complete meal, serve with a cooked vegetable, such as broccoli, or with sliced fresh tomatoes.*

Potato pancakes are best when served hot right from the pan!

Tips

For extra convenience, use 2 cups (500 mL) grated hash-brown potatoes, available at the supermarket. Use the fresh (not frozen) variety with no added fat. Put the hash browns in a microwave-safe bowl, cover with plastic wrap and microwave on High for 3 to 4 minutes, until just tender. Let cool to room temperature before adding other ingredients.

Pair these with Homemade Turkey Sausage (see recipe, page 39).

Exchanges Per Serving

| 3 | Starch |
| 1 1/2 | Fat |

Nutrient Analysis Per Serving

Calories	342
Protein	9 g
Fat	11 g
Saturated fat	2 g
Carbohydrate	51 g
Fiber	5 g
Cholesterol	109 mg
Sodium	631 mg

Corn on the Cob

For the best corn on the cob, it is important to use the freshest corn — and don't overcook it!

Tip

To determine freshness when buying corn, look for silk that is still green and moist and kernels that are in uniform rows and aren't too large.

6	medium cobs of corn, husks and silks removed	6

Flavored Butter

3 tbsp	butter, softened, or soft margarine	45 mL
½ tsp	salt	2 mL
¼ tsp	freshly ground black pepper	1 mL
1 tbsp	minced green onion	15 mL
	or	
1 tbsp	chopped fresh parsley	15 mL
	or	
½ tsp	chili powder	2 mL
	or	
2 tbsp	freshly grated Parmesan cheese	30 mL

1. In a large pot of boiling salted water, cook corn over medium heat for about 5 minutes, or until corn is tender.
2. *Meanwhile, prepare the flavored butter:* Combine butter with salt, pepper and your choice of green onion, parsley, chili powder or Parmesan cheese.
3. Drain corn and serve with flavored butter.

Dietitian's Message *Serve vegetables you know your kids will eat. Most kids love raw baby carrots or carrot sticks, snow peas, raw "broccoli trees," sliced cucumber and corn on the cob.*

Exchanges Per Serving

1	Starch
1½	Fat

Nutrient Analysis Per Serving

Calories	139
Protein	4 g
Fat	8 g
Saturated fat	1 g
Carbohydrate	18 g
Fiber	3 g
Cholesterol	2 mg
Sodium	310 mg

Mexican Corn

2 cups	frozen corn kernels	500 mL
1 tbsp	butter	15 mL
1/4 cup	diced cooking onions	50 mL
1/4 cup	diced green bell peppers	50 mL
1/4 cup	diced red bell peppers	50 mL
1/2 tsp	salt	2 mL
1/4 tsp	freshly ground black pepper	1 mL

1. Place corn in a medium microwave-safe dish, cover and microwave on High for 4 to 5 minutes, until hot.

2. Meanwhile, in a small saucepan, melt butter over medium heat. Add onions and green and red peppers and cook for 2 to 3 minutes, or until softened. Stir into corn, add salt and pepper and serve.

Dietitian's Message *Brightly colored vegetables, such as corn and red and green bell peppers, are good sources of antioxidants, such as beta carotene, and other phytochemicals, as well as fiber. It's a good idea to eat a variety of vegetables every day. Five to 10 servings of fruits and vegetables are recommended daily.*

For a complete Mexican meal, serve with Refrito Quesadillas (see recipe, page 120) or Soft Chicken Tacos (see recipe, page 116).

Tip

To steam vegetables in the microwave: Cover the dish with plastic wrap (not wax paper), and do not add water. There is enough moisture on freshly washed or frozen vegetables to steam them. Be careful when you remove the plastic wrap, because the steam is very hot even if the dish isn't. If you aren't using the vegetables right away, plunging them in ice-cold water will help them retain their bright color.

Exchanges Per Serving

1	Starch
1/2	Fat

Nutrient Analysis Per Serving

Calories	108
Protein	3 g
Fat	4 g
Saturated fat	2 g
Carbohydrate	20 g
Fiber	2 g
Cholesterol	8 mg
Sodium	305 mg

Zucchini Boats

Don't overcook these "boats" — they look and taste better if the zucchini is cooked only until tender-crisp.

- Preheat oven to 350°F (180°C)
- 9-inch (2.5 L) square baking dish

1	clove garlic, minced	1
¼ cup	diced onions	50 mL
2	medium zucchini (about 1 lb/500 g)	2
2	medium tomatoes, seeded and diced	2
2 tbsp	lower-fat Italian dressing	25 mL
¼ cup	freshly grated Parmesan cheese	50 mL
2 tbsp	cooked bacon bits	25 mL

Tip

You can also barbecue these boats. It's best to use a covered barbecue with a shelf above the main grilling rack. Place stuffed zucchini boats on a sheet of foil on the shelf 4 inches (10 cm) above the grill and cook with the barbecue lid closed for 10 to 15 minutes, until heated through and the cheese is melted.

Variation

Substitute an equal amount of feta or Cheddar cheese for the Parmesan.

1. Place garlic and onions in a small microwave-safe dish, cover and microwave on High for 1 minute, or until onion is softened.

2. Cut zucchini in half lengthwise and scoop out the flesh, leaving a ½-inch (1 cm) shell. Place the zucchini shells in baking dish. Cut the scooped-out flesh into small cubes.

3. In a medium bowl, combine zucchini cubes, tomatoes and onion mixture. Spoon evenly into hollowed zucchini shells. Drizzle with Italian dressing and sprinkle with Parmesan and bacon bits.

4. Bake in preheated oven for 15 to 20 minutes, or until vegetables are tender and cheese is melted.

Dietitian's Message

Here's a great way to make vegetables kid-friendly! Sprinkling the zucchini boats and their contents with Parmesan and bacon bits creates a whole new, delicious taste.

Exchanges Per Serving

1	Vegetable
½	Lean Meat
½	Fat

Nutrient Analysis Per Serving

Calories	80
Protein	5 g
Fat	4 g
Saturated fat	2 g
Carbohydrate	8 g
Fiber	3 g
Cholesterol	5 mg
Sodium	283 mg

Sandwiches, Burgers and Pizzas

Chicken Caesar Wraps

Try this recipe with tortillas of different colors and flavors.

Tip

Avocados turn brown quickly. Brushing the exposed slices with lemon juice slows the discoloration — and in this recipe the lemon enhances the flavor.

4	leaves romaine lettuce	4
4	8-inch (20 cm) flour tortillas	4
2½ cups	cooked diced chicken breasts (about 8 oz/250 g)	625 mL
½ cup	diced tomato (about 1 medium)	125 mL
8	thin slices red onion	8
1	avocado, sliced (10 oz/300 g)	1
1 tsp	freshly squeezed lemon juice	5 mL
1	clove garlic, minced	1
¼ cup	lower-fat mayonnaise	50 mL

1. Lay a lettuce leaf on each tortilla. In the center of each lettuce leaf, place equal portions of chicken, tomato and onion.

2. Brush avocado slices with lemon juice. Layer on top of the onion.

3. In a small bowl, stir together garlic and mayonnaise. Drizzle over chicken and vegetables.

4. Tucking in one end of the tortillas, roll each one up as tightly as possible and serve.

Dietitian's Message *Here's a fun way to eat a sandwich — just wrap it! The avocado is chock full of healthy monounsaturated fat. Why not try this for lunch soon?*

Exchanges Per Serving

1	Starch
2	Vegetable
2	Lean Meat
1½	Fat

Nutrient Analysis Per Serving

Calories	332
Protein	21 g
Fat	15 g
Saturated fat	2 g
Carbohydrate	29 g
Fiber	3 g
Cholesterol	48 mg
Sodium	290 mg

BLT Wraps

4	8-inch (20 cm) flour tortillas	4
3 oz	lower-fat cream cheese (about 6 tbsp/90 mL)	90 g
8 oz	lean cooked ham, sliced	250 g
8	leaves leaf lettuce	8
2	medium tomatoes, diced	2
2 tbsp	fat-free ranch dressing	25 mL
¼ cup	cooked bacon bits	50 mL

1. Spread each tortilla with 1½ tbsp (20 mL) cream cheese. Cover with ¼ of the ham. Place 2 lettuce leaves on top of the ham and arrange ¼ of the diced tomato down the center of each tortilla. Drizzle with ½ tbsp (7 mL) ranch dressing and sprinkle with 1 tbsp (15 mL) bacon bits. Roll up the tortillas, tucking in one end so the filling stays intact.

Wraps make a nice change from sandwiches in lunch boxes and at picnics.

Tip

The best way to cook bacon in the microwave is to place 4 slices between 2 or 3 folded paper towels. Microwave on High for 3 to 4 minutes. The paper towel soaks up the excess fat and makes cleanup easy!

Exchanges Per Serving

1	Starch
1	Vegetable
2	Lean Meat
1	Fat

Nutrient Analysis Per Serving

Calories	304
Protein	18 g
Fat	13 g
Saturated fat	4 g
Carbohydrate	25 g
Fiber	2 g
Cholesterol	43 mg
Sodium	1235 mg

*Whip up these hot
and tasty deli melts
for a gang of hungry
teens or use mini
bagels as a base and
make a platter of
party snacks.*

Tip

Substitute your
favorite lean deli meat.
Roast beef, corned
beef, ham and turkey
are almost identical
in terms of fat content.

Open-Face Deli Melts

- *Baking sheet*

1	medium onion, sliced	1
1	green bell pepper, sliced	1
2 tbsp	fat-free ranch dressing	25 mL
2	bagels (each 3 oz/90 g), split in half	2
2 tsp	Dijon mustard	10 mL
8 oz	sliced cooked deli turkey, ham or lean beef	250 g
½ cup	shredded Swiss cheese	125 mL

1. Preheat broiler with the oven rack 4 to 5 inches (10 to 13 cm) from the element.
2. Place onion and pepper in a small microwave-safe dish; cover and microwave on Medium-High (70%) for about 3 minutes, or until tender-crisp, stirring halfway through. Drain and toss with ranch dressing.
3. Spread bagel halves with mustard, top with sliced meat and sprinkle with Swiss.
4. Place bagels on baking sheet and broil for 3 minutes, until cheese is melted.
5. Top each sandwich with hot onion mixture and serve.

Dietitian's Message

When tasty food is easy to make, older kids and teens will get into the action. Keep a variety of cold cuts and bagels on hand for a hearty and nutritious lunch or snack. This beats the endless trips to the cupboard at snack time for chips, cookies and crackers.

Exchanges Per Serving

1½ Starch

1 Vegetable

2 Lean Meat

Nutrient Analysis Per Serving

Calories	263
Protein	20 g
Fat	7 g
Saturated fat	3 g
Carbohydrate	30 g
Fiber	2 g
Cholesterol	37 mg
Sodium	981 mg

Tuna Melts on Pitas

Tuna melts are an old favorite, updated on a lower-fat pita.

- *Baking sheet*

¼ cup	lower-fat mayonnaise, divided	50 mL
6	6-inch (15 cm) pitas	6
2	cans (each 7½ oz/213 g) flaked water-packed tuna, drained	2
2	dill pickles, chopped	2
¼ cup	chopped celery	50 mL
¼ cup	minced green onions	50 mL
1 cup	shredded lower-fat Cheddar cheese	250 mL

1. Preheat broiler with the oven rack 4 to 5 inches (10 to 13 cm) from the element.

2. Spread 1 tsp (5 mL) of the mayonnaise on each pita.

3. In a small bowl, combine tuna, pickles, celery, green onions and the remaining 2 tbsp (25 mL) mayonnaise. Spread tuna mixture over the pitas and sprinkle evenly with Cheddar.

4. Place on baking sheet and broil for 3 minutes, until cheese is hot and bubbling.

Tip

Always choose water-packed tuna. A 3-oz (90 g) serving of water-packed tuna has only 1 gram of fat; the same amount of oil-packed tuna has 8 to 12 grams of fat.

Dietitian's Message

Teens can make this as an after-school or bedtime snack on a hungry and active day. It's easy to make and sure to satisfy. It's nutritious, with protein and carbohydrate, but very low in fat.

Exchanges Per Serving

2	Starch
1	Vegetable
2	Lean Meat

Nutrient Analysis Per Serving

Calories	328
Protein	24 g
Fat	8 g
Saturated fat	3 g
Carbohydrate	38 g
Fiber	2 g
Cholesterol	34 mg
Sodium	775 mg

Picnic Hero

You'll be the hero when you produce this giant Dagwood sandwich!

Tips

When you can't find ripe tomatoes, try this trick to ripen tomatoes at home. Put unripened tomatoes into a brown paper bag with an apple. Poke a few holes in the bag and keep at room temperature for 2 to 3 days.

Keep it safe: when transporting food for a picnic, be sure to pack your food in a tightly sealed ice-packed cooler. Remember to always keep cold food cold and hot food hot!

Exchanges Per Serving

2	Starch
1	Vegetable
2	Lean Meat and Meat Substitute
1	Fat

Nutrient Analysis Per Serving

Calories	315
Protein	22 g
Fat	12 g
Saturated fat	4 g
Carbohydrate	38 g
Fiber	3 g
Cholesterol	34 mg
Sodium	1251 mg

Mustard Spread

1 tbsp	Dijon mustard	15 mL
1 tbsp	lower-fat mayonnaise	15 mL
1 tbsp	lower-fat sour cream	15 mL
½ tsp	prepared horseradish	2 mL

Sandwich

1	loaf (12 oz/375 g) French bread	1
2	dill pickles, thinly sliced	2
12	lettuce leaves	12
10 oz	thinly sliced cooked deli turkey	300 g
4	slices processed Swiss cheese	4
2	medium tomatoes, thinly sliced	2
½	red onion, thinly sliced	½
1 cup	alfalfa sprouts	250 mL
3 tbsp	lower-fat mayonnaise	45 mL

1. *Prepare the mustard spread:* In a small bowl, combine mustard, mayonnaise, sour cream and horseradish.

2. *Prepare the sandwich:* Cut bread in half lengthwise and spread mustard spread on the bottom half. Layer on pickles, lettuce and turkey. Cut Swiss cheese in half diagonally and arrange on top of the turkey. Layer on tomatoes, red onion and alfalfa sprouts. Spread mayonnaise on the top half of the bread and close the sandwich.

3. Cut sandwich into 6 slices to serve, or wrap well and refrigerate for up to 4 hours. Slice just before serving.

Meatball Subs

*Yummy and runny!
Have lots of napkins
handy when you serve
these subs.*

Barbecue Sauce

1 tsp	vegetable oil	5 mL
1/4 cup	chopped onions	50 mL
1/4 cup	chopped green bell peppers	50 mL
1	can (7.5 oz/213 mL) tomato sauce	1
3 tbsp	ketchup	45 mL
2 tbsp	packed brown sugar	25 mL
2 tbsp	red wine vinegar	25 mL
1/2 tsp	Worcestershire sauce	2 mL

Meatballs

1	large egg	1
1 lb	lean ground beef	500 g
2 tbsp	dry bread crumbs	25 mL
2 tbsp	minced onion	25 mL
1/2 tsp	salt	2 mL
1/2 tsp	garlic powder	2 mL
1/2 tsp	Worcestershire sauce	2 mL
1/4 tsp	freshly ground black pepper	1 mL
6	small submarine or hero buns (each 2 oz/60 g)	6

Tips

Egg and bread crumbs
help bind ground
meat together so
it won't crumble
while cooking.

Meatballs can be made
in advance, covered
and refrigerated for up
to 2 days or frozen in
an airtight container
for up to 2 months.

1. *Prepare the barbecue sauce:* In a medium saucepan, heat oil over medium-high heat. Add onions and peppers and sauté for 2 minutes, until softened. Add tomato sauce, ketchup, brown sugar, vinegar and Worcestershire sauce; reduce heat and simmer, uncovered, for 15 minutes, until slightly thickened.

2. *Prepare the meatballs:* In a medium bowl, combine egg, ground beef, bread crumbs, onion, salt, garlic powder, Worcestershire sauce and pepper and mix well. Using a heaping teaspoon (5 mL) for each, shape into 24 meatballs.

3. Preheat a large nonstick skillet, sprayed with vegetable spray, over medium-high heat. Add meatballs and fry, stirring often, for 5 to 6 minutes, until brown on all sides and no longer pink inside.

4. Cut buns in half and place 4 meatballs on the bottom half of each bun. Spoon hot barbecue sauce over the meatballs, cover with the top half of the bun and serve.

**Exchanges
Per Serving**

2	Starch
1/2	Other Carbohydrate
2	Vegetable
1	Medium-Fat Meat
1 1/2	Fat

**Nutrient Analysis
Per Serving**

Calories	421
Protein	22 g
Fat	17 g
Saturated fat	6 g
Carbohydrate	46 g
Fiber	1 g
Cholesterol	78 mg
Sodium	903 mg

The egg and tuna fillings can also be served on lettuce greens for a low-carbohydrate main dish salad.

Tip

Eggshells are difficult to remove from very fresh eggs after they are hard-cooked. As eggs become older, they are easier to peel, so use the oldest eggs in your fridge for hard-cooking.

Exchanges Per Serving

2	Starch
1	Vegetable
1	Medium-Fat Meat
1 1/2	Fat

Nutrient Analysis Per Serving

Calories	348
Protein	15 g
Fat	15 g
Saturated fat	3 g
Carbohydrate	38 g
Fiber	1 g
Cholesterol	221 mg
Sodium	612 mg

Salad Bar Subs

Light Egg Salad Subs

Egg Salad

4	large eggs, hard-cooked and cooled	4
2	small green onions, sliced	2
1/4	green bell pepper, diced	1/4
2 tbsp	lower-fat mayonnaise	25 mL
1 tsp	Dijon mustard (optional)	5 mL
	Salt and freshly ground black pepper	
4	small submarine buns (each 2 oz/60 g)	4
2 tbsp	lower-fat mayonnaise	25 mL
8	lettuce leaves	8
1	large tomato, thinly sliced	1
1/2	cucumber, thinly sliced	1/2
1 cup	alfalfa sprouts	250 mL
4	slices bacon, cooked	4

1. *Prepare the egg salad:* In a small bowl, chop eggs. Add green onions, green pepper, mayonnaise and mustard, if using, and combine. Season with salt and pepper to taste.

2. Slice each bun in half and spread both halves with mayonnaise. Arrange lettuce on the bottom half. Dividing the ingredients equally among the four buns, spoon on egg salad and top with tomato, cucumber, alfalfa sprouts and bacon. Cover with the top half of the buns.

Tuna Egg Salad Subs

Tuna Salad

1	can (7.5 oz/213 g) water-packed tuna, drained	1
1	large egg, hard-cooked and cooled	1
2	small green onions, sliced	2
2 tbsp	grated carrot	25 mL
2 tbsp	lower-fat mayonnaise	25 mL
4	small submarine buns (2 oz/60 g each)	4
2 tbsp	lower-fat mayonnaise	25 mL
8	lettuce leaves	8
1	large tomato, thinly sliced	1
½	cucumber, thinly sliced	½
1 cup	alfalfa sprouts	250 mL
4	slices bacon, cooked	4

1. *Prepare the tuna salad:* In a medium bowl, flake tuna with a fork. Chop the egg and stir into the tuna, along with green onions, grated carrot and mayonnaise.

2. Slice each bun in half and spread both halves with mayonnaise. Arrange lettuce on the bottom half. Dividing the ingredients equally among the four buns, spoon on tuna egg salad and top with tomato, cucumber, alfalfa sprouts and bacon. Cover with the top half of the buns.

> **Dietitian's Message** *Parents and kids are always looking for ideas for school lunches. Stuff these fillings into pitas for a change. With a fruit and milk or yogurt, it is a complete meal.*

Exchanges Per Serving

2	Starch
1	Vegetable
2	Lean Meat
1	Fat

Nutrient Analysis Per Serving

Calories	339
Protein	21 g
Fat	12 g
Saturated fat	2 g
Carbohydrate	37 g
Fiber	1 g
Cholesterol	77 mg
Sodium	568 mg

Kids can impress their friends at a campfire cookout by serving "gourmet" wiener kabobs!

Tip

When cooking at a campfire, you need long skewers for these kabobs so you can keep away from the hot coals. Be cautious, and use oven mitts when using metal skewers, as the handles get hot too!

Variation

Substitute 8 oz (250 g) cubed ham or cooked sausage for the wieners. Serve with potato salad and coleslaw or on submarine buns with mustard and ketchup, if desired.

Exchanges Per Serving

2 Vegetable

1½ Fat

Nutrient Analysis Per Serving

Calories	141
Protein	6 g
Fat	9 g
Saturated fat	4 g
Carbohydrate	10 g
Fiber	2 g
Cholesterol	23 mg
Sodium	448 mg

Hot Dog Kabobs

- *Four 14-inch (35 cm) metal skewers*

4	all-beef wieners	4
1	green bell pepper, cut into 1-inch (2.5 cm) pieces	1
½ cup	pineapple chunks (drained, if canned)	125 mL
4	cherry tomatoes	4
¼ cup	barbecue sauce (store-bought or see recipe, page 91)	50 mL

1. Cut the hot dogs into 5 pieces each. Alternately thread wiener pieces, pepper and pineapple chunks onto skewers. Top each skewer with a cherry tomato. Brush lightly with barbecue sauce.

2. Grill over hot coals for about 15 minutes, until lightly browned.

Dietitian's Message *There are now a variety of wieners available, including tofu and turkey wieners. Tofu wieners, being made from soybeans, are cholesterol-free and a source of protein, vitamin E, calcium, iron and zinc. Serve vegetarian tofu wieners for a change.*

Turkey-Mozza Burgers

You can make a big juicy burger that is low in fat thanks to the lean ground turkey.

- *Preheat barbecue*

1	large egg	1
¼ cup	minced green onions (optional)	50 mL
¼ cup	minced parsley (optional)	50 mL
2 tbsp	dry bread or cracker crumbs	25 mL
1 tsp	Dijon mustard	5 mL
1 tsp	salt	5 mL
½ tsp	garlic powder	2 mL
½ tsp	dried basil	2 mL
1 lb	lean ground turkey or chicken	500 g
1 cup	shredded part-skim mozzarella cheese	250 mL
6	hamburger or Kaiser buns (each 1½ oz/45 g)	6

1. In a medium bowl, mix together egg, green onions (if using), parsley (if using), bread crumbs, 2 tbsp (25 mL) water, mustard, salt, garlic and basil. Using your hands, mix in ground turkey and shape into 6 patties about ¾ inch (2 cm) thick.

2. Barbecue patties (or fry in a lightly greased nonstick skillet) for about 7 minutes per side, until internal temperature has reached 175°F (80°C) and burgers are no longer pink inside. Top with mozzarella and cook for 1 minute, until cheese melts.

3. Serve on buns with your choice of toppings (see suggestions in tip, at left).

Dietitian's Message

Burgers are always popular with children and teens because they can be eaten without utensils. Use whole wheat hamburger or Kaiser buns, as well as tomatoes and lettuce, to pump up the fiber content.

Tip

Be sure to thoroughly wash your hands and the preparation area with lots of soap after touching raw poultry.

Great toppings for burgers that don't add a lot of carbohydrates or calories are: lettuce or spinach leaves, tomato slices, thinly sliced onions (grilled, sautéed or raw), cooked sliced mushrooms, dill pickle slices, sauerkraut.

Variation

Serve burgers wrapped in pitas instead of on buns.

Exchanges Per Serving

1½	Starch
3	Lean Meat
½	Fat

Nutrient Analysis Per Serving

Calories	319
Protein	24 g
Fat	13 g
Saturated fat	5 g
Carbohydrate	25 g
Fiber	0 g
Cholesterol	109 mg
Sodium	805 mg

Teriyaki Burgers

The chopped water chestnuts add a nice crunchiness to Japanese-style burgers.

Tip

As a general rule, 4 oz (125 g) raw meat yields 3 oz (90 g) cooked.

- Preheat barbecue

I	large egg	I
I lb	lean ground beef	500 g
I cup	chopped water chestnuts	250 mL
2 tbsp	dry bread crumbs	25 mL
I	clove garlic, minced	I
¼ cup	soy sauce	50 mL
2 tbsp	sliced green onion	25 mL
2 tbsp	granulated sugar	25 mL
½ tsp	ground ginger	2 mL
8	slices canned pineapple, packed in juice, drained (optional)	8
4	crusty hamburger buns (1½ oz/45 g each)	4

1. In a medium bowl, combine egg, ground beef, water chestnuts and bread crumbs. Shape into 4 patties about ¾ inch (2 cm) thick and place in a shallow dish.

2. In a small bowl, combine garlic, soy sauce, green onion, sugar and ginger. Pour over hamburger patties, cover and refrigerate for at least 1 hour or overnight.

3. Barbecue the patties (or fry in a lightly greased nonstick skillet) for 7 minutes, flip, brush with marinade and barbecue for 7 to 8 minutes more, or until internal temperature has reached 170°F (75°C) and burgers are no longer pink inside.

4. Top each patty with 2 pineapple slices, if desired, and serve on buns.

Exchanges Per Serving

2 Starch
½ Other Carbohydrate
3½ Lean Meat
½ Fat

Nutrient Analysis Per Serving

Calories	436
Protein	32 g
Fat	15 g
Saturated fat	6 g
Carbohydrate	40 g
Fiber	I g
Cholesterol	122 mg
Sodium	1321 mg

Potato Chip Fish (page 109) ▶
Overleaf: Chicken Fajita Salad (page 75)

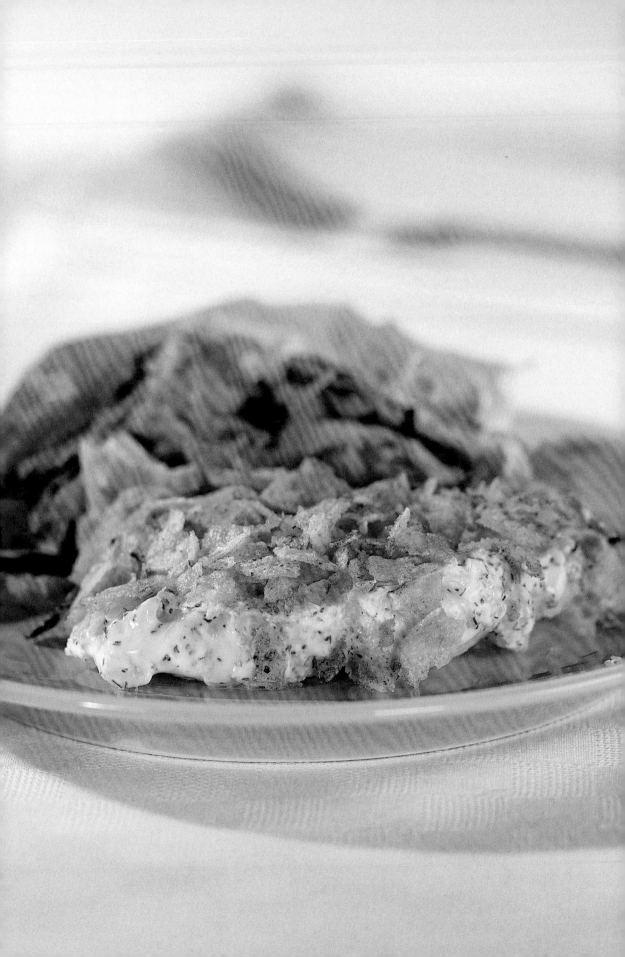

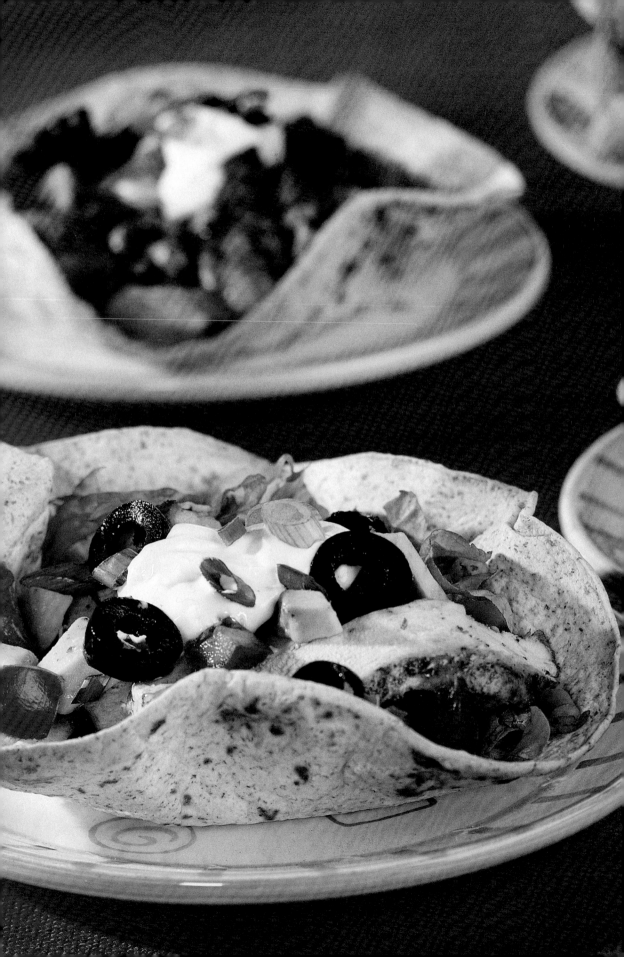

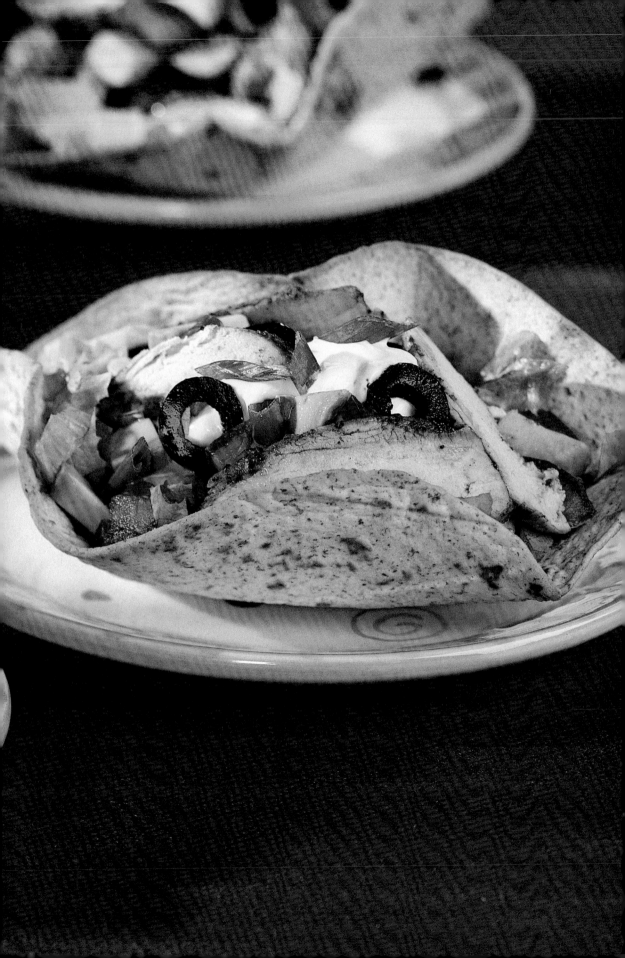

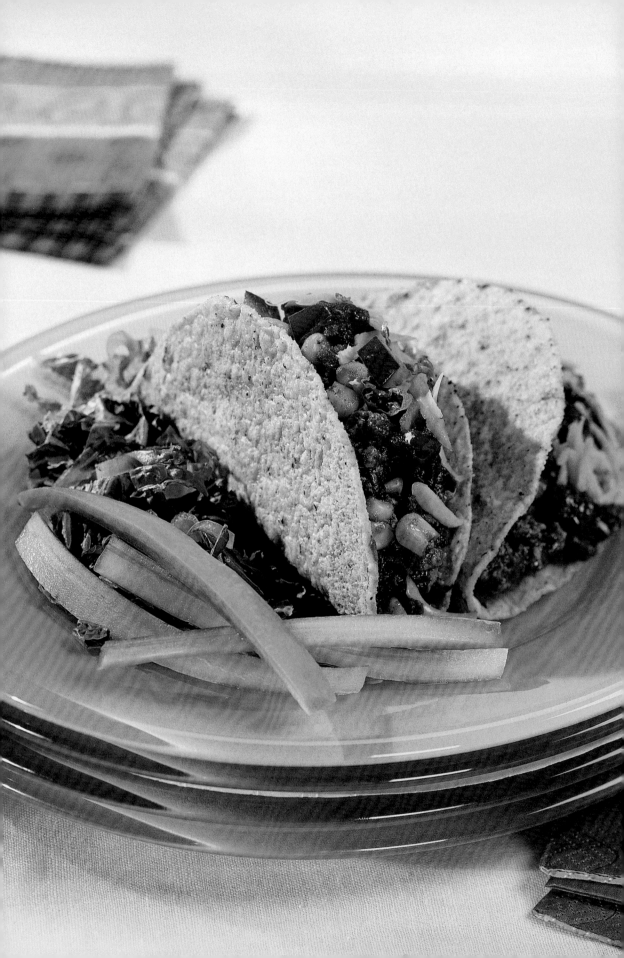

Chili Burgers

These messy burgers are great camping fare!

- *Preheat barbecue*

I tsp	vegetable oil	5 mL
I	clove garlic, minced	I
½ cup	chopped onions	125 mL
¼ cup	chopped green bell peppers	50 mL
I ½ cups	canned vegetarian chili with beans	375 mL
I ¼ lb	lean ground beef	625 g
6	hamburger buns (each I½ oz/45 g)	6
I ½ cups	shredded lettuce	375 mL
I cup	shredded lower-fat Cheddar cheese	250 mL
12	slices green bell pepper	12
6	slices onion	6

Variation

Use wieners and hot dog buns to make chili cheese dogs!

1. In a medium saucepan, heat oil over medium-high heat. Add garlic, onions and green peppers and cook, stirring, for 2 to 3 minutes, until softened. Add chili and let simmer while you prepare the burgers.

2. Shape ground beef into 6 patties about ¾ inch (2 cm) thick. Barbecue (or fry in a lightly greased nonstick skillet) for about 7 minutes per side, or until internal temperature has reached 170°F (75°C) and burgers are no longer pink inside.

3. Toast hamburger buns, if desired.

4. For each burger, divide about ½ the shredded lettuce evenly among the bottom half of the buns and top with a hamburger patty, ¼ cup (50 mL) chili mixture, 3 tbsp (45 mL) Cheddar, green pepper and onion slices, remaining lettuce and the top half of the bun.

Dietitian's Message *With chili beans, ground beef and Cheddar cheese, these burgers are loaded with protein. Even the hungriest teens will find these filling. Serve with fruit salad and a glass of milk to round out the nutrients.*

◀ Tex's Tacos (page 117)

Exchanges Per Serving

2	Starch
4	Medium-Fat Meat

Nutrient Analysis Per Serving

Calories	469
Protein	35 g
Fat	21 g
Saturated fat	10 g
Carbohydrate	34 g
Fiber	3 g
Cholesterol	80 mg
Sodium	788 mg

Fillet of Fish Burgers

Tips

Great toppings that don't add a lot of carbohydrates or calories are: lettuce or spinach leaves, tomato slices, thinly sliced onions (grilled, sautéed or raw), dill pickle slices.

White fish fillets are very similar in terms of taste and nutrition, so choose what you like — but remember that fresh is always best, so be flexible and pick what is in season.

Exchanges Per Serving

1½ Starch

2½ Very Lean Meat

½ Fat

Nutrient Analysis Per Serving

Calories	250
Protein	21 g
Fat	7 g
Saturated fat	2 g
Carbohydrate	26 g
Fiber	2 g
Cholesterol	36 mg
Sodium	390 mg

- *Preheat oven to 425°F (220°C)*
- *Baking sheet, sprayed with vegetable spray*

1 lb	skinless white fish fillets (cod, halibut or sole)	500 g
2	egg whites	2
1 tbsp	vegetable oil	15 mL
½ cup	corn flakes cereal crumbs	125 mL
¼ cup	freshly grated Parmesan cheese	50 mL
6	crusty whole wheat buns (each 1½ oz/45 g) or pitas	6
6 tbsp	Light Tartar Sauce (see recipe, facing page)	90 mL

1. Cut fish fillets into 6 equal pieces.

2. In a shallow dish, using a fork, beat egg whites and oil.

3. In a separate shallow dish, combine corn flakes crumbs and Parmesan. Dip fish pieces first into egg mixture, then into crumbs. Press crumbs on to make sure they stick. Discard any excess egg and crumb mixtures.

4. Place fish on prepared baking sheet and bake in preheated oven for 18 to 20 minutes, or until coating is golden brown and fish flakes easily when tested with a fork. Don't overcook.

5. Serve on whole wheat buns, topped with 1 tbsp (15 mL) Light Tartar Sauce and your choice of toppings (see suggestions in tip, at left).

> **Dietitian's Message** *Breads baked from whole-grain flours contain more vital nutrients than more refined breads. Encourage your family to choose whole wheat in recipes such as this one.*

Light Tartar Sauce

½ cup	plain yogurt	125 mL
⅓ cup	lower-fat mayonnaise	75 mL
3 tbsp	chopped dill pickle	45 mL
I tsp	freshly squeezed lemon juice	5 mL
½ tsp	Dijon mustard	2 mL
Dash	hot pepper sauce	Dash
Dash	Worcestershire sauce	Dash

Tip
This recipe can be
stored in a well-sealed
container (or a jar with
a tight-fitting lid) in
the refrigerator for up
to 5 days.

I. In a small bowl, stir together yogurt, mayonnaise,
   pickles, lemon juice, mustard, hot pepper sauce and
   Worcestershire sauce. Cover and refrigerate for at least
   2 hours, until completely chilled and flavors are
   blended. Serve with fish or on fish burgers.

**Exchanges
Per Serving**

Free Food

**Nutrient Analysis
Per Serving**

Calories	19
Protein	0 g
Fat	I g
Saturated fat	0 g
Carbohydrate	I g
Fiber	0 g
Cholesterol	0 mg
Sodium	71 mg

Tuna Burgers

Tuna burgers are perfect for camping or picnics — instead of baking them, make them early in the day, wrap them in foil and keep cold, and barbecue them later.

Tip

To hard-cook eggs, place eggs in a saucepan and cover with cold water. Heat to boiling, then reduce heat to medium-low and simmer for 10 minutes. Run eggs under cold water to stop cooking.

• *Preheat oven to 350°F (180°C)*

1	large egg, hard-cooked	1
1	large egg white, hard-cooked	1
1 tbsp	minced green onion	15 mL
1 tbsp	minced green bell pepper	15 mL
1 tbsp	minced dill pickle	15 mL
1	can (7½ oz/213 g) water-packed tuna, drained	1
1 cup	shredded lower-fat Cheddar cheese	250 mL
¼ cup	lower-fat mayonnaise	50 mL
4	hamburger buns (each 1½ oz/45 g)	4

1. In a medium bowl, chop hard-boiled egg and egg white. Mix in green onion, green pepper and pickle.

2. Flake tuna with a fork. Add to the egg mixture, along with Cheddar and mayonnaise. Stir gently until well combined.

3. Divide mixture into four equal portions and spread on the bottom half of the buns. Replace the top of the buns and wrap in foil.

4. Bake in preheated oven for 20 minutes, until heated through. Unwrap carefully and serve.

Dietitian's Message *Two non-meat meals a week (including fish) are recommended for a healthy diet. When canned tuna is packed in water, rather than oil, the fat content is much lower. Tuna is a good source of omega-3 fatty acids, which are healthy fats.*

Exchanges Per Serving

1½ Starch

2½ Lean Meat

1 Fat

Nutrient Analysis Per Serving

Calories	325
Protein	23 g
Fat	14 g
Saturated fat	5 g
Carbohydrate	25 g
Fiber	0 g
Cholesterol	116 mg
Sodium	592 mg

French Bread Pizza

- *Broiler pan*

I	small loaf French bread (about 8 oz/250 g)	I
2 cups	sliced mushrooms	500 mL
2	green onions, sliced	2
I	tomato, diced	I
½ cup	chopped green bell peppers	125 mL
2 cups	shredded part-skim mozzarella cheese	500 mL
I cup	chopped pepperoni or ham (about 4 oz/125 g)	250 mL
½ cup	pizza or pasta sauce	125 mL

1. Preheat broiler and position oven rack 5 to 6 inches (13 to 15 cm) from the element. Cut French bread in half lengthwise, place on broiler pan, cut side up, and toast lightly under the broiler.

2. In a small microwave-safe bowl, covered with plastic wrap with one corner turned back, microwave mushrooms on High for 2 minutes, or until softened.

3. In a medium bowl, combine mushrooms, green onions, tomato and green peppers. Add mozzarella and pepperoni and toss lightly to mix.

4. Spread pizza sauce on toasted bread and spoon on toppings.

5. Broil for 3 to 4 minutes, or until cheese is melted. Cut into 4 pieces and serve.

MAKES 4 SERVINGS

French bread makes a lovely, crispy base for quick pizzas.

Variations

Chicken Fajita Pizza Bread: Substitute salsa for the pizza sauce, cooked chicken for the pepperoni, and Monterey Jack for the mozzarella. Omit the mushrooms and add 1 diced red bell pepper.

Greek Pizza Bread: Omit the pepperoni and mushrooms. Add ½ cup (125 mL) sliced black olives and 8 oz (250 g) cooked small shrimp. Substitute crumbled feta for ⅔ cup (150 mL) of the mozzarella.

Exchanges Per Serving

2	Starch
2	Vegetable
3	Medium-Fat Meat
2	Fat

Nutrient Analysis Per Serving

Calories	506
Protein	27 g
Fat	26 g
Saturated fat	11 g
Carbohydrate	42 g
Fiber	3 g
Cholesterol	57 mg
Sodium	1362 mg

Use this pizza dough as the base for the delicious recipes on pages 103–106.

Tip

If you are not going to make pizzas immediately, brush the balls of dough with vegetable oil, wrap loosely in plastic wrap and refrigerate for up to 12 hours. When ready to make pizzas, let dough stand at room temperature for 15 minutes before rolling out into pizza rounds.

Easy Pizza Dough

1	envelope (¼ oz/7 g) instant yeast	1
1½ cups	all-purpose flour	375 mL
¾ cup	whole wheat flour	175 mL
1 tsp	salt	5 mL
½ tsp	granulated sugar	2 mL
¾ cup	hot water	175 mL

1. In a food processor — or in a large bowl, using a wooden spoon — mix together yeast, all-purpose flour, whole wheat flour, salt and sugar. Add water and process or stir until the dough forms a ball (if you need more water, add it 1 tbsp/15 mL at a time). Process for 1 minute or knead by hand for 3 to 4 minutes, until dough is smooth and elastic. Cover dough loosely with plastic wrap and let rise for 10 minutes.

2. Divide dough into 6 pieces for individual pizzas or into 2 balls for a large pizza.

**Exchanges
Per Serving**

2	Starch

**Nutrient Analysis
Per Serving**

Calories	172
Protein	6 g
Fat	1 g
Saturated fat	0 g
Carbohydrate	36 g
Fiber	3 g
Cholesterol	0 mg
Sodium	387 mg

SANDWICHES, BURGERS AND PIZZAS

Sloppy Joe Pizza

- Preheat oven to 400°F (200°C)
- Large baking sheet or pizza pans, sprinkled lightly with cornmeal

8 oz	lean ground beef	250 g
1	clove garlic, minced	1
½ cup	chopped onions	125 mL
¾ cup	pizza or pasta sauce	175 mL
½ tsp	chili powder	2 mL
Pinch	salt	Pinch
Pinch	freshly ground black pepper	Pinch
	Easy Pizza Dough (see recipe, page 102)	
1½ cups	shredded part-skim mozzarella cheese	375 mL

1. In a large nonstick skillet, over medium heat, cook ground beef for 3 minutes, stirring occasionally. Add garlic and onions and continue cooking for about 5 minutes, until meat is browned and crumbly and onion is softened. Stir in pizza sauce, chili powder, salt and pepper.

2. On a clean work surface, with lightly buttered fingers or a rolling pin, spread dough into six 5- to 6-inch (13 to 15 cm) rounds or two 10-inch (25 cm) rounds on prepared baking sheet. Spread with meat sauce and sprinkle with mozzarella.

3. Bake in preheated oven for 15 to 20 minutes, until cheese is melted and crust is golden brown. Let cool for 5 minutes before cutting and serving.

MAKES 6 SERVINGS

Sloppy Joe Pizza is sloppy, so make sure to supply lots of napkins!

Variation

For a meatless version, substitute vegetarian ground soy meat alternative for the ground beef.

Exchanges Per Serving

2	Starch
2	Vegetable
2	Lean Meat
1	Fat

Nutrient Analysis Per Serving

Calories	382
Protein	22 g
Fat	13 g
Saturated fat	6 g
Carbohydrate	44 g
Fiber	4 g
Cholesterol	41 mg
Sodium	692 mg

Taco Pizza

- *Preheat oven to 400°F (200°C)*
- *Large baking sheet or pizza pans, sprinkled lightly with cornmeal*

8 oz	lean ground turkey	250 g
½ cup	chopped onions	125 mL
2½ tbsp	taco seasoning mix	32 mL
	Easy Pizza Dough (see recipe, page 102)	
1½ cup	shredded part-skim mozzarella cheese	375 mL

1. In a large nonstick skillet, over medium heat, cook ground turkey for 3 minutes, stirring occasionally. Add onions and cook for 3 to 4 minutes, until meat is browned and crumbly and onion is softened. Add taco seasoning and ¼ cup (50 mL) water; bring to a boil. Reduce heat to low and simmer, uncovered, for 10 minutes, until thickened.

2. On a clean work surface, with lightly buttered fingers or a rolling pin, spread dough into six 5- to 6-inch (13 to 15 cm) rounds or two 10-inch (25 cm) rounds on prepared baking sheet. Spread with taco meat and sprinkle with mozzarella.

3. Bake in preheated oven for 15 to 20 minutes, until cheese is melted and crust is golden brown. Let cool for 5 minutes before cutting and serving.

4. Serve with toppings of your choice (see suggestions in tip, at left).

Exchanges Per Serving

2½ Starch

2 Lean Meat

Nutrient Analysis Per Serving

Calories	318
Protein	20 g
Fat	9 g
Saturated fat	4 g
Carbohydrate	40 g
Fiber	4 g
Cholesterol	47 mg
Sodium	626 mg

Funny Face Pizza

- *Preheat oven to 400°F (200°C)*
- *Large baking sheet or pizza pans, sprinkled lightly with cornmeal*

	Easy Pizza Dough (see recipe, page 102)	
2 cups	pizza or pasta sauce	500 mL
2 cups	shredded part-skim mozzarella cheese	500 mL
2 oz	pepperoni (12 slices)	60 g
1	green bell pepper, sliced	1
8	black olives	8
1 cup	grated carrots	250 mL

1. Divide dough into 8 balls and spread into 4- to 5-inch (10 to 13 cm) rounds on prepared baking sheet. Spread with pizza sauce and sprinkle with mozzarella. Arrange pepperoni, green pepper and olives on top of the cheese to look like funny faces: cut pepperoni slices in half to use for mouth and eyes; green peppers become ears and eyebrows; an olive makes the nose.

2. Bake in preheated oven for 15 to 20 minutes, until cheese is melted and crust is golden brown. Let cool for 5 minutes before cutting and serving.

3. Garnish each pizza with grated carrots for hair.

Variation

Make monstrous funny face pizzas for Halloween.

Exchanges Per Serving

1½	Starch
2	Vegetable
1	Medium-Fat Meat
1½	Fat

Nutrient Analysis Per Serving

Calories	356
Protein	16 g
Fat	15 g
Saturated fat	6 g
Carbohydrate	41 g
Fiber	5 g
Cholesterol	27 mg
Sodium	1053 mg

Virtuous Veggie Pizza

Tips

If stewed tomatoes are not available in 14-oz (398 mL) cans, substitute a 19-oz (540 mL) can, keeping in mind that the nutrient analysis will change slightly.

Stewed tomatoes sometimes have large chunks. If desired, after draining, transfer tomatoes to a cutting board and chop into smaller pieces.

- *Preheat oven to 400°F (200°C)*
- *Large baking sheet or pizza pans, sprinkled lightly with cornmeal*

I	red or green bell pepper, chopped	I
2 cups	broccoli florets	500 mL
I cup	sliced carrots and/or zucchini	250 mL
I cup	sliced mushrooms	250 mL
	Easy Pizza Dough (see recipe, page 102)	
2 cups	shredded part-skim mozzarella cheese	500 mL
I	can (14 oz/398 mL) Italian-style stewed tomatoes, drained (see tips, at left)	I
2 tbsp	grated Parmesan cheese	25 mL

1. In a large microwave-safe bowl, covered with plastic wrap with one corner turned back, microwave red pepper, broccoli, carrots and mushrooms on High for 2 to 3 minutes, or until tender-crisp. Rinse under cold water and drain.

2. On a clean work surface, with lightly buttered fingers or a rolling pin, spread dough into six 5- to 6-inch (13 to 15 cm) rounds or two 10-inch (25 cm) rounds on prepared baking sheet. Sprinkle with 1 cup (250 mL) mozzarella, top with drained tomatoes and cooked vegetables, then sprinkle with the remaining 1 cup (250 mL) mozzarella and Parmesan.

3. Bake in preheated oven for 15 to 20 minutes, until cheese is melted and crust is golden brown. Let cool for 5 minutes before cutting and serving.

Exchanges
Per Serving

2	Starch
2	Vegetable
I	Medium-Fat Meat

Nutrient Analysis
Per Serving

Calories	334
Protein	19 g
Fat	8 g
Saturated fat	5 g
Carbohydrate	49 g
Fiber	6 g
Cholesterol	25 mg
Sodium	803 mg

Dietitian's Message *Loaded with antioxidants and phytochemicals, this veggie pizza is indeed virtuous. Broccoli is a source of flavonoids, and tomatoes have lycopene; both help to protect against cancers. Red bell peppers have carotenoids, which are antioxidants.*

Dinners

White fish fillets are mild-flavored and dry out easily when cooking. This crunchy coating adds flavor and seals in moistness.

Tip

Testing for doneness: When cooking fish fillets or steaks, pierce with a fork in the thickest part. The flesh should flake easily and should be opaque throughout.

Exchanges
Per Serving

1	Starch
4	Very Lean Meat
1½	Fat

Nutrient Analysis Per Serving

Calories	284
Protein	31 g
Fat	11 g
Saturated fat	2 g
Carbohydrate	15 g
Fiber	2 g
Cholesterol	65 mg
Sodium	486 mg

Crunchy Peanut Fish Fillets

- Preheat oven to 425°F (220°C)
- Baking sheet, sprayed with vegetable spray

1 cup	dry bread crumbs	250 mL
½ cup	dry-roasted peanuts	125 mL
1 tsp	dried parsley	5 mL
½ tsp	salt	2 mL
½ tsp	freshly ground black pepper	2 mL
3 tbsp	lower-fat mayonnaise	45 mL
1 tsp	freshly squeezed lime juice	5 mL
1½ lb	skinless sole fillets (or other white fish)	750 g

1. In a food processor, combine bread crumbs, peanuts, parsley, salt and pepper and process until finely chopped. Pour into a shallow dish.

2. In another shallow dish, combine mayonnaise and lime juice. Coat fish fillets with the mayonnaise mixture, then dip into crumb mixture, pressing gently so that crumbs stick to both sides. Place on prepared baking sheet. Discard any excess mayonnaise and crumb mixtures.

3. Bake in preheated oven for 6 minutes. Turn and bake for 3 to 4 minutes more, or until coating is crispy and fish is opaque throughout and flakes easily when pierced with a fork.

Dietitian's Message *Almost all fish are low in fat, and the fat they do contain is rich in beneficial omega-3 fatty acids. Fish is also a great convenience food, delicious and quick-cooking. Children often enjoy the milder taste and delicate texture of sole in recipes such as this one. Why not choose fish for dinner more often?*

Potato Chip Fish

- *Preheat oven to 425°F (220°C)*
- *Baking sheet, sprayed with vegetable spray*

I	clove garlic, minced	I
¼ cup	plain yogurt	50 mL
I tsp	dried dillweed	5 mL
I tsp	freshly squeezed lemon juice	5 mL
I lb	skinless cod fillets (or other white fish)	500 g
I	bag (1½ oz/42 g) potato chips, crushed (about ½ cup/125 mL crushed chips)	

1. In a small bowl, combine garlic, yogurt, dill and lemon juice.
2. Divide fillets into 4 pieces of equal size and place on prepared baking sheet. Spread with yogurt mixture and sprinkle with crushed potato chips.
3. Bake in preheated oven for 12 to 15 minutes, or until topping is golden brown and fish flakes easily when pierced with a fork.

Dietitian's Message *This is an amazing combination, encouraging kids to eat fish with one of their favorite foods, potato chips. The lower-fat fish helps to balance the fat in the chips.*

The crispy chip topping will be a hit with the whole family.

Variations

Try different flavors of potato chips, such as dill pickle, sour cream and onion or salt and vinegar.

Substitute 4 small skinless boneless chicken breasts for the fish fillets and increase baking time to 25 to 30 minutes.

Exchanges Per Serving

½ Starch
3 Very Lean Meat

Nutrient Analysis Per Serving

Calories	160
Protein	22 g
Fat	5 g
Saturated fat	1 g
Carbohydrate	7 g
Fiber	0 g
Cholesterol	49 mg
Sodium	69 mg

Everybody loves fish sticks — why not make your own?

Fish Sticks

- Preheat oven to 425°F (220°C)
- Baking sheet, sprayed with vegetable spray

1 lb	skinless firm white fish fillets (cod or halibut)	500 g
³⁄₄ cup	dry whole wheat bread crumbs	175 mL
¹⁄₄ cup	cornmeal	50 mL
¹⁄₂ tsp	salt	2 mL
¹⁄₄ tsp	freshly ground black pepper	1 mL
¹⁄₄ tsp	ground dried thyme	1 mL
1	large egg	1
2 tbsp	lower-fat ranch dressing	25 mL
	Light Tartar Sauce (see recipe, page 99) or ketchup	

1. Cut fish crosswise into 12 sticks.

2. In a shallow dish, combine bread crumbs, cornmeal, salt, pepper and thyme.

3. In another shallow dish, beat egg with a fork. Stir in ranch dressing and beat until well combined.

4. Dip fish sticks in egg mixture, then roll in crumbs, pressing gently so that crumbs stick to both sides. Arrange on prepared baking sheet and sprinkle with any remaining crumbs. Discard any excess egg.

5. Bake in preheated oven for 12 to 15 minutes, or until topping is golden brown and fish flakes easily when pierced with a fork. Serve with Light Tartar Sauce or ketchup.

Exchanges Per Serving

¹⁄₂	Starch
3	Very Lean Meat
¹⁄₂	Fat

Nutrient Analysis Per Serving

Calories	191
Protein	24 g
Fat	5 g
Saturated fat	1 g
Carbohydrate	12 g
Fiber	1 g
Cholesterol	105 mg
Sodium	445 mg

Dietitian's Message *Eggs are good sources of protein, vitamins and minerals. Egg yolks contain fat and cholesterol that egg whites do not. Whole eggs are recommended for children because there is some iron in the yolks, and most kids do not need to be concerned about cholesterol and fat.*

Salmon Croquettes

1	can (7½ oz/213 g) sockeye salmon	1
1	large egg	1
¼ cup	dry bread crumbs	50 mL
2 tbsp	lower-fat mayonnaise	25 mL
¼ tsp	salt	1 mL
¼ tsp	freshly ground black pepper	1 mL
¼ tsp	freshly squeezed lemon juice	1 mL
2 tsp	vegetable oil	10 mL
	Light Tartar Sauce (see recipe, page 99)	

These tasty fish cakes are a quick dinner solution — just use that can of salmon you have stored in the pantry.

Tip

Just for fun, on Valentine's Day make heart-shaped salmon croquettes and serve with pink Fettuccini Alfredo (see recipe, page 128; add pink food coloring to the sauce).

1. Drain salmon. Place in a small bowl and mash with a fork, including bones and skin. Add egg, bread crumbs, mayonnaise, salt, pepper and lemon juice and mix gently until blended. Form into 8 small patties about ½ inch (1 cm) thick and place on a plate. Cover with waxed paper and refrigerate for at least 30 minutes or for up to 6 hours.

2. In a large nonstick skillet, heat oil over medium heat. Add patties and fry for 8 to 10 minutes per side, turning only once, until golden and heated through.

3. Serve hot with Light Tartar Sauce.

Dietitian's Message *When fish is not well liked by children, serving it croquette-style may do the trick. Not only does it not look like fish, but the crispy pan-fried breading adds a nice flavor that kids like.*

Exchanges Per Serving

½	Starch
1½	Lean Meat
1	Fat

Nutrient Analysis Per Serving

Calories	173
Protein	11 g
Fat	11 g
Saturated fat	2 g
Carbohydrate	6 g
Fiber	0 g
Cholesterol	67 mg
Sodium	471 mg

Provide lots of napkins — this finger food is sticky!

Tip

Marinades usually have acidic ingredients that may react with the dish they are marinated in. Never marinate meat in a metal dish unless it is stainless steel. An easy way to marinate foods is to place the meat and the marinade in a freezer bag with a seal; this makes it easy to mix occasionally too.

Exchanges
Per Serving

1	Other Carbohydrate
2½	Medium-Fat Meat
½	Fat

Nutrient Analysis
Per Serving

Calories	271
Protein	19 g
Fat	16 g
Saturated fat	4 g
Carbohydrate	13 g
Fiber	0 g
Cholesterol	76 mg
Sodium	721 mg

Orange-Glazed Chicken Wings

• *Baking sheet, lined with foil and sprayed with vegetable spray*

12	chicken wings, tips removed (about 1 lb/500 g)	12
¼ cup	orange juice concentrate	50 mL
¼ cup	soy sauce	50 mL
2 tbsp	liquid honey	25 mL
½ tsp	ground ginger	2 mL
½ tsp	garlic powder	2 mL

1. Place chicken wings in a non-reactive (glass, plastic or stainless steel) bowl.

2. In a small bowl, combine orange juice concentrate, soy sauce, honey, ginger and garlic powder. Mix well and pour over the wings. Cover and refrigerate for at least 1 hour or for up to 8 hours. Meanwhile, preheat oven to 375°F (190°C).

3. Remove wings from marinade, reserving extra marinade. Arrange wings on prepared baking sheet. Bake in preheated oven for 20 minutes.

4. After wings have baked for 20 minutes, turn and brush with reserved marinade. Continue baking for 20 minutes, or until juices run clear when wings are pierced with a fork.

Dietitian's Message *Chicken wings tend to be high in fat because there is more skin for the amount of meat. For an occasional treat, however, they make a great appetizer or part of a meal. Try balancing the fat by consuming lower-fat foods in the rest of the meal or over the course of the day.*

Oven-Baked Crispy Chicken

A moist and crispy fried chicken taste without the fat of traditional fried chicken.

- Preheat oven to 350°F (180°C)
- Baking sheet, sprayed with vegetable spray

4	chicken leg quarters (about 1 lb/500 g)	4
½ cup	corn flakes cereal crumbs	125 mL
2 tbsp	freshly grated Parmesan cheese	25 mL
2 tsp	garlic powder	10 mL
2 tsp	seasoning salt	10 mL
2 tsp	chili powder	10 mL
½ tsp	freshly ground black pepper	2 mL
¼ cup	1% milk	50 mL

1. Rinse chicken and remove all skin and visible fat. Pat dry. Cut apart at the joint into thighs and drumsticks.

2. In a large plastic bag, combine corn flakes crumbs, Parmesan, garlic powder, seasoning salt, chili powder and pepper.

3. Pour milk into a shallow dish.

4. Dip chicken pieces in milk, then add them, one at a time, to the plastic bag. Shake to coat with crumbs. Place on prepared baking sheet and sprinkle with any remaining crumbs. Discard any excess milk.

5. Bake in preheated oven for 45 to 50 minutes, or until juices run clear when chicken is pierced with a fork.

Tip

Removing the skin from chicken cuts the fat by more than half.

Dietitian's Message *The carbohydrate count in this recipe is minimal compared to the appetite satisfaction. Team with Smashed Potatoes (see recipe, page 77) and Zucchini Boats (see recipe, page 84).*

Exchanges Per Serving

1 Starch

3½ Lean Meat

Nutrient Analysis Per Serving

Calories	232
Protein	29 g
Fat	6 g
Saturated fat	2 g
Carbohydrate	13 g
Fiber	1 g
Cholesterol	107 mg
Sodium	840 mg

*Serve chicken fingers
as a dinner entrée
or as part of a
party platter with
your choice of
dipping sauce.*

Variation

Substitute 1 cup
(250 mL) crushed
crisp rice cereal for
the crackers and cut
chicken into chunks
instead of strips to
make nuggets.

**Exchanges
Per Serving**

1	Starch
½	Other Carbohydrate
2½	Lean Meat

**Nutrient Analysis
Per Serving**

Calories	242
Protein	23 g
Fat	7 g
Saturated fat	1 g
Carbohydrate	21 g
Fiber	0 g
Cholesterol	53 mg
Sodium	581 mg

Chicken Fingers with Dipping Sauces

- *Preheat oven to 400°F (200°C)*
- *Baking sheet, sprayed with vegetable spray*

24	soda crackers	24
¼ cup	lower-fat mayonnaise	50 mL
1 lb	skinless boneless chicken breasts (about 4)	500 g
	Plum Dipping Sauce or Honey Mustard Sauce (see recipes, facing page)	

1. In a food processor, process soda crackers (or place in a plastic bag and crush with a rolling pin into fine crumbs). Pour into a shallow dish.

2. Spoon mayonnaise into another shallow dish.

3. Rinse chicken and pat dry with paper towels. Using a sharp knife, cut each breast lengthwise into 6 strips.

4. Add strips to mayonnaise and turn to coat evenly. Roll the coated strips, one at a time, in cracker crumbs and arrange in a single layer on prepared baking sheet. Discard any excess mayonnaise and crumbs.

5. Bake in preheated oven for 15 minutes, turn and bake for 10 to 15 minutes more, or until coating is crisp and golden and chicken is no longer pink inside.

6. Serve with Plum Dipping Sauce and/or Honey Mustard Sauce.

Plum Dipping Sauce

3 tbsp	bottled plum sauce	45 mL
1 tbsp	ketchup	15 mL
2 tsp	soy sauce	10 mL
1 tsp	vinegar	5 mL

1. In a small bowl, combine plum sauce, ketchup, soy sauce and vinegar.

Honey Mustard Sauce

3 tbsp	Dijon mustard	45 mL
1 tbsp	liquid honey	15 mL
1 tbsp	fat-free sour cream	15 mL

1. In a small bowl, combine Dijon mustard, honey and sour cream.

Soft Chicken Tacos

These are very messy tacos, so you're well advised to eat them with a knife and fork rather than trying to pick them up!

Tips

It's easier to cut meat into strips if it is partially frozen: slice it before it is completely thawed. If it is already thawed, place it in the freezer for 30 minutes before slicing.

You can find taco seasoning mix in bulk food dispensers at the grocery store. For this recipe, you could instead use half of a 1¼ oz (35 g) package.

Exchanges Per Serving

2½ Starch
2 Vegetable
3 Lean Meat
1½ Fat

Nutrient Analysis Per Serving

Calories	506
Protein	34 g
Fat	18 g
Saturated fat	7 g
Carbohydrate	50 g
Fiber	3 g
Cholesterol	74 mg
Sodium	689 mg

- Preheat oven to 350°F (180°C)

12 oz	skinless boneless chicken breasts (about 3)	375 g
1 tsp	vegetable oil	5 mL
1	medium onion, diced	1
2½ tbsp	taco seasoning mix	32 mL
8	8-inch (20 cm) flour tortillas	8
1	medium tomato, diced	1
1 cup	shredded lettuce	250 mL
1 cup	shredded Monterey Jack cheese	250 mL
½ cup	salsa (store-bought or see recipe, page 58)	125 mL
½ cup	fat-free sour cream	125 mL

1. Cut chicken breasts into thin strips lengthwise along the grain of the meat.

2. In a large nonstick skillet, heat oil over medium-high heat. Add chicken strips and stir-fry for 5 to 6 minutes, or until no longer pink inside. Add onion and continue to stir-fry for 1 minute. Add taco seasoning and ½ cup (125 mL) water. Bring to a boil, then reduce heat to low and simmer for 10 minutes, until thickened.

3. Meanwhile, wrap tortillas in foil. Warm in preheated oven for 10 minutes. Remove from oven and unwrap, being careful of the steam.

4. Spoon hot chicken onto the tortillas and top with tomato, lettuce, Monterey Jack, salsa and sour cream. Fold tacos in half and serve.

Tex's Tacos

- *Preheat oven to 350°F (180°C)*
- *Baking sheet, ungreased*

1 lb	lean ground turkey	500 g
2	cloves garlic, minced	2
½ cup	chopped onions	125 mL
1 cup	drained and rinsed chickpeas or kidney beans	250 mL
½ cup	frozen corn kernels	125 mL
¼ cup	ketchup	50 mL
2 tbsp	chili powder	25 mL
1 tsp	salt	5 mL
10	hard taco shells	10
1	large tomato, diced	1
2 cups	shredded lettuce	500 mL
1¼ cups	shredded lower-fat Cheddar cheese	300 mL
⅓ cup	salsa (store-bought or see recipe, page 58)	75 mL

These tacos taste great and are loaded with healthy fiber. They are also a little spicy, so if you don't like spicy food, reduce the amount of chili powder and use mild salsa.

1. In a large nonstick skillet, over medium-high heat, cook ground turkey for 5 to 6 minutes, or until browned and crumbly. Add garlic and onions and cook for 2 to 3 minutes, or until onions are softened.

2. In a small bowl, mash chickpeas with a fork or potato masher until coarsely mashed. Add to the turkey mixture, with corn, ketchup, ¼ cup (50 mL) water, chili powder and salt. Simmer for 10 minutes, stirring occasionally, until thickened.

3. Meanwhile, place taco shells on baking sheet and bake in preheated oven for 7 to 10 minutes, until crisp and light golden brown.

4. Spoon meat mixture into taco shells and top with tomato, lettuce, Cheddar and salsa.

Dietitian's Message *This recipe is a balanced meal. All the food groups are represented, and the chickpeas boost the healthy fiber.*

Exchanges Per Serving

1½	Starch
2	Vegetable
3	Lean Meat
1½	Fat

Nutrient Analysis Per Serving

Calories	421
Protein	30 g
Fat	17 g
Saturated fat	4 g
Carbohydrate	39 g
Fiber	6 g
Cholesterol	78 mg
Sodium	992 mg

Garden Burritos

These easy burritos contain cilantro, a member of the parsley family. Not everyone likes it, so leave it out if it's not to your taste.

Variation

Add 1 cup (250 mL) chopped cooked turkey, chicken, pork or roast beef.

- Preheat oven to 400°F (200°C)
- 13- by 9-inch (3 L) baking pan, sprayed with vegetable spray

1	can (19 oz/540 mL) black beans, drained and rinsed	1
1	can (14 oz/398 mL) kernel corn, drained	1
1	can (14 oz/398 mL) Mexican-style stewed tomatoes	1
1½ cups	shredded Monterey Jack cheese	375 mL
1 tbsp	chopped fresh cilantro	15 mL
8	8-inch (20 cm) flour tortillas	8

1. In a medium bowl, combine beans, corn, tomatoes, Monterey Jack and cilantro.

2. Lay tortillas out and divide bean mixture evenly in the center of the tortillas. Fold the bottom end up over the filling, tuck the sides in and roll up.

3. Place burritos, fold side down, in prepared baking pan. Bake in preheated oven for 10 minutes, until burritos are heated through and cheese is melted.

Dietitian's Message *Here's another great meatless recipe! Serve each baked burrito with salad and a glass of milk. Finish with Cherry Cobbler (see recipe, page 173).*

Exchanges Per Serving

2½ Starch

1 Medium-Fat Meat

½ Fat

Nutrient Analysis Per Serving

Calories	323
Protein	15 g
Fat	10 g
Saturated fat	5 g
Carbohydrate	46 g
Fiber	7 g
Cholesterol	19 mg
Sodium	529 mg

Chili Con Carne

12 oz	extra-lean ground beef	375 g
1	clove garlic, minced	1
¼ cup	diced onions	50 mL
¼ cup	chopped green bell peppers	50 mL
1	can (19 oz/540 mL) kidney beans, drained and rinsed	1
1	can (14 oz/398 mL) diced tomatoes	1
1 tbsp	chili powder	15 mL
1 tbsp	unsweetened cocoa powder	15 mL
1 tbsp	granulated sugar	15 mL
1 tbsp	white vinegar	15 mL
1 tsp	pumpkin pie spice	5 mL
½ tsp	salt	2 mL

Cocoa and pumpkin pie spice are the secret ingredients in this chili.

Tip

If your kids don't like onions, substitute ½ tsp (2 mL) onion powder for the diced onions.

Variation

Serve chili on rice, pasta, french fries or a baked potato, topped with shredded Cheddar cheese and fat-free sour cream.

1. Heat a large saucepan over medium-high heat. Add ground beef and cook for 5 to 7 minutes, stirring often, until browned and crumbly.

2. Add garlic, onions and green peppers and cook, stirring, for 2 to 3 minutes, until garlic is fragrant and onions begin to soften. Stir in kidney beans, tomatoes, chili powder, cocoa, sugar, vinegar, pumpkin pie spice and salt. Increase heat to high and bring to a boil.

3. Reduce heat to low and simmer for at least 30 minutes or for up to 1 hour to allow flavors to blend. Add ¼ cup (50 mL) water if chili becomes too thick.

Dietitian's Message *Kidney beans are an excellent source of both soluble and insoluble fiber, containing 6 grams per ½-cup (125 mL) serving. Most people get only half of the 25 to 35 grams of fiber they need daily. Children need an amount of fiber that equals their age plus 5 grams.*

Exchanges Per Serving

1½	Starch
2	Vegetable
3	Lean Meat
½	Fat

Nutrient Analysis Per Serving

Calories	400
Protein	28 g
Fat	14 g
Saturated fat	5 g
Carbohydrate	43 g
Fiber	11 g
Cholesterol	48 mg
Sodium	589 mg

Refrito Quesadillas

Quesadillas are good for lunches or snacks, and they make a great party platter when cut into smaller wedges and arranged with small bowls of salsa and sour cream.

Tip

Quesadillas are traditionally fried, but baking them works well and cuts down on fat. Don't try to reheat them in the microwave, though, as they will lose their nice crispy texture.

- Preheat oven to 350°F (180°C)
- Baking sheet, ungreased

2	cloves garlic, minced	2
½ cup	diced onions	125 mL
¼ cup	diced red or green bell peppers	50 mL
1	can (14 oz/398 mL) refried beans	1
1 tbsp	minced jalapeño pepper (optional)	15 mL
1 tsp	chili powder	5 mL
¼ tsp	ground cumin (optional)	1 mL
6	8-inch (20 cm) flour tortillas	6
1½ cups	shredded part-skim mozzarella cheese	375 mL
2	green onions, chopped	2
	Salsa (store-bought or see recipe, page 58)	
	Fat-free sour cream (optional)	

1. In a medium saucepan, over medium heat, cook garlic, onions and peppers until garlic is fragrant and onions soften, about 3 minutes. Stir in refried beans, jalapeño pepper (if using), chili powder and cumin (if using); cook for 10 to 15 minutes, until slightly thickened and vegetables are softened. Let cool to room temperature.

2. Arrange 3 tortillas in a single layer on baking sheet. Divide bean mixture evenly among the 3 tortillas and spread almost to edges, sprinkle with mozzarella and green onions and top with the 3 remaining tortillas. Bake for 15 to 20 minutes, or until tortillas are golden and cheese is melted.

3. Cut each quesadilla into 6 wedges and serve with salsa and fat-free sour cream, if desired.

Dietitian's Message *Read the ingredient list of refried beans carefully — they may contain lard. Make your brand choice carefully to avoid getting unwanted fat. Lard is a saturated fat and is considered heart-unhealthy.*

Exchanges
Per Serving

1½ Starch
1 Vegetable
2½ Medium-Fat Meat

Nutrient Analysis
Per Serving

Calories	360
Protein	23 g
Fat	14 g
Saturated fat	8 g
Carbohydrate	35 g
Fiber	5 g
Cholesterol	44 mg
Sodium	669 mg

Hawaiian Chili

1 tsp	vegetable oil	5 mL
1 lb	lean ground turkey	500 g
1	clove garlic, minced	1
1/4 cup	diced onions	50 mL
1/4 cup	diced green bell peppers	50 mL
1	can (19 oz/540 mL) kidney beans, drained and rinsed	1
1	can (14 oz/398 mL) stewed tomatoes	1
1	can (5 1/2 oz/156 mL) tomato paste	1
3 tbsp	soy sauce	45 mL
2 tsp	chili powder	10 mL
2 tsp	packed brown sugar	10 mL
3 cups	cooked long-grain white rice	750 mL
1/4 cup	chopped green onions	50 mL

1. In a large saucepan, heat oil over medium-high heat. Add ground turkey and cook for 6 to 8 minutes, stirring often, until browned and crumbly. Add garlic, onions and green peppers and cook for 2 to 3 minutes, until garlic is fragrant and onions begin to soften.

2. Stir in kidney beans, tomatoes, tomato paste, soy sauce, chili powder and brown sugar and bring to a boil. Reduce heat to medium-low and simmer for at least 30 minutes or for up to 1 hour to allow flavors to blend. If chili becomes too thick, add 1/4 cup (50 mL) water.

3. For each serving, spread 1/2 cup (125 mL) rice on a dinner plate, top with 1 cup (250 mL) chili and sprinkle with green onions.

Dietitian's Message *This is a delicious chili, and it's so healthy! Try using brown rice instead of white for more fiber, and increase the water and cooking time according to package directions. For a vegetarian meal, substitute 12 oz (375 g) vegetarian ground soy meat alternative for the ground turkey.*

I first tasted this satisfying combination of chili and rice several years ago, after a hard day of waterskiing in Hawaii.

Tip

When cooking lean ground meat, it is usually necessary to brown it in a bit of vegetable oil to prevent it from sticking and burning. Medium ground meat usually has enough fat to prevent it from sticking without extra oil. If using medium, drain off any excess fat before adding remaining ingredients.

Exchanges Per Serving

2 1/2	Starch
2	Vegetable
2	Lean Meat

Nutrient Analysis Per Serving

Calories	389
Protein	25 g
Fat	7 g
Saturated fat	2 g
Carbohydrate	57 g
Fiber	8 g
Cholesterol	60 mg
Sodium	737 mg

Lasagna

Variation

Substitute whole wheat
or spinach lasagna
noodles, or cut down
on preparation time by
using no-boil lasagna
noodles, which are
widely available at
grocery stores.

**Exchanges
Per Serving**

2	Starch
2	Vegetable
3½	Lean Meat
½	Fat

**Nutrient Analysis
Per Serving**

Calories	425
Protein	29 g
Fat	13 g
Saturated fat	5 g
Carbohydrate	49 g
Fiber	3 g
Cholesterol	70 mg
Sodium	689 mg

- Preheat oven to 350°F (180°C)
- 13- by 9-inch (3 L) baking dish or lasagna pan

1 tsp	olive oil	5 mL
8 oz	lean ground turkey or beef	250 g
2	cloves garlic, minced	2
1	onion, diced	1
½	green bell pepper, diced	½
1	can (14 oz/398 mL) diced or crushed tomatoes	1
1	can (5½ oz/156 mL) tomato paste	1
8 oz	mushrooms, sliced (about 3 cups/750 mL)	250 g
2 tsp	dried Italian seasoning	10 mL
½ tsp	salt	2 mL
½ tsp	freshly ground black pepper	2 mL
12	lasagna noodles	12
3	green onions, chopped	3
1	large egg	1
2 cups	1% cottage cheese	500 mL
2 cups	shredded part-skim mozzarella cheese, divided	500 mL
2 tbsp	freshly grated Parmesan cheese	25 mL

1. In a large nonstick skillet, heat olive oil over medium-high heat. Add ground turkey and cook for 6 to 8 minutes, or until browned and crumbly.

2. Add garlic, onion and green pepper and cook, stirring, for 2 to 3 minutes, until onions are softened. Stir in tomatoes, tomato paste, mushrooms, Italian seasoning, salt and pepper. Bring to a boil, then reduce heat to low and simmer for 30 minutes to allow flavors to blend.

3. Meanwhile, boil lasagna noodles according to package instructions until tender to the bite; do not overcook. Drain, rinse with cold water to stop cooking and set aside.

4. In a small bowl, combine green onions, egg and cottage cheese.

5. Spread a little meat sauce in the bottom of the baking dish. Top with 4 cooked noodles, overlapping slightly, Top with $\frac{1}{2}$ of the cottage cheese mixture and $\frac{1}{3}$ of the meat sauce. Sprinkle with $\frac{2}{3}$ cup (150 mL) of the mozzarella.

6. Repeat the layers (4 noodles, remaining cottage cheese, $\frac{1}{3}$ of the meat sauce, $\frac{2}{3}$ cup/150 mL mozzarella). Top with the remaining 4 noodles, remaining meat sauce and Parmesan cheese.

7. Cover with foil and bake in preheated oven for 40 minutes. Remove foil, sprinkle with the remaining $\frac{2}{3}$ cup (150 mL) mozzarella and bake, uncovered, for 10 minutes, until cheese is melted and lasagna is hot and bubbling around the edges. Let cool for 10 minutes before serving.

Dietitian's Message *Lasagna is an all-time favorite for most kids, and it's full of healthy foods: starch, protein, dairy, vegetables. It allows you to sneak vegetables into your kids' diets in a way they won't protest. For a meatless version, substitute vegetarian ground soy meat alternative for the turkey or beef.*

Lazy Lasagna

This fast and easy dinner has all the flavors of traditional baked lasagna and is ready in a fraction of the time.

Variation

For a meatless version, substitute vegetarian ground soy meat alternative for the ground turkey.

8 oz	wide egg noodles	250 g
12 oz	lean ground turkey	375 g
1	jar (24 oz/700 mL) traditional pasta sauce	1
1	package (10 oz/300 g) frozen chopped spinach, thawed, excess liquid squeezed out	1
1	large egg	1
1½ cups	1% cottage cheese	375 mL
1¼ cups	shredded part-skim mozzarella cheese	300 mL
¼ cup	freshly grated Parmesan cheese	50 mL

1. Cook egg noodles in a large pot of boiling salted water following package instructions until tender to the bite. Drain.

2. Meanwhile, heat a large, deep nonstick skillet, sprayed with vegetable spray, over medium-high heat. Add ground turkey and cook for 5 to 6 minutes, stirring often, until browned and crumbly. Transfer to a large bowl and combine with tomato sauce.

3. In another large bowl, stir together spinach, egg and cottage cheese.

4. Spread ⅓ of the tomato-meat sauce over the bottom of the skillet. Evenly arrange ⅓ of the cooked noodles over the sauce and spread with ½ of the cottage cheese mixture. Spoon another ⅓ of the sauce over the cottage cheese and top with another ⅓ of the noodles. Spread with the remaining cottage cheese mixture and sprinkle with shredded mozzarella. Arrange remaining noodles on top and cover with the remaining sauce.

Exchanges Per Serving

2½ Starch

2 Vegetable

2½ Lean Meat

½ Fat

Nutrient Analysis Per Serving

Calories	434
Protein	36 g
Fat	14 g
Saturated fat	6 g
Carbohydrate	42 g
Fiber	4 g
Cholesterol	143 mg
Sodium	1178 mg

5. Cover the pan and bring to a boil over medium-high heat. Reduce heat to medium-low and simmer for 15 minutes, until hot and bubbly. Sprinkle with Parmesan, remove from heat and let stand for 5 minutes before serving.

Dietitian's Message *When purchasing ground turkey, check that the label says "ground turkey breast." Some ground turkey does not contain only breast meat, and the fat content will be higher.*

Lasagna Roll-ups

These roll-ups look fancy, but they are easy to make. You can use homemade or store-bought pasta sauce, or stuff the filling into no-boil cannelloni for an even easier meal.

Variations

Add 2 cups (500 mL) cooked chopped shrimp to the cottage cheese filling.

Substitute a 10-oz (300 g) package of frozen chopped spinach for the broccoli. Thaw it and drain completely by placing in a colander and squeezing out all excess moisture with the back of a spoon.

Exchanges
Per Serving

3	Starch
4	Vegetable
2	Lean Meat
1/2	Fat

Nutrient Analysis
Per Serving

Calories	496
Protein	29 g
Fat	12 g
Saturated fat	5 g
Carbohydrate	68 g
Fiber	4 g
Cholesterol	56 mg
Sodium	1073 mg

- *Preheat oven to 350°F (180°C)*
- *13- by 9-inch (3 L) baking dish*

12	lasagna noodles	12
1	package (10 oz/300 g) frozen chopped broccoli	1
2	green onions, chopped	2
1	large egg	1
2 cups	1% cottage cheese	500 mL
1/4 cup	freshly grated Parmesan cheese	50 mL
1/2 tsp	salt	2 mL
2 cups	pasta sauce	500 mL
1 cup	shredded part-skim mozzarella cheese	250 mL

1. In a large pot of boiling salted water, cook lasagna noodles according to package directions until tender to the bite. Drain and rinse with cold water to stop cooking.

2. Meanwhile, in a medium microwave-safe dish, covered with plastic wrap with one corner turned back, microwave broccoli on High for 3 minutes until completely thawed. Add green onions and continue cooking for 1 minute, until onions are softened. Rinse immediately under cold water to retain bright green color. Drain well.

3. In a medium bowl, combine egg, cottage cheese, Parmesan and salt. Stir in cooked broccoli and green onions.

4. Place cooked noodles on waxed paper. Spread broccoli-cheese mixture evenly on the noodles and roll up jelly-roll style.

5. Spread ⅔ of the spaghetti sauce in the bottom of the baking dish. Arrange rolled noodles, seam side down, on the sauce. Top with remaining sauce and cover with foil.

6. Bake in preheated oven for 25 minutes. Uncover, sprinkle with mozzarella and continue baking for 10 minutes, until cheese is melted and rolls are heated through.

Dietitian's Message *Here's a meatless dish that's easy to make and will please the whole family. Remember, meatless meals are recommended as a main course at least twice a week.*

This is a much lighter version of a classic family favorite. You can make it with dried pasta, but it tastes better if you use fresh pasta.

Tip

What is the yield of dried pasta after cooking? For long types, such as spaghetti, linguini and fettuccine, 2 oz (60 g) dried (or a bundle ½ inch/1 cm in diameter) yields 1 cup (250 mL) cooked al dente. For short types, such as macaroni, rotini or shells, 2 oz (60 g) dried (or just over ½ cup/250 mL) yields 1 cup (250 mL) cooked.

Exchanges Per Serving

2	Starch
1	Lean Meat

Nutrient Analysis Per Serving

Calories	234
Protein	12 g
Fat	6 g
Saturated fat	3 g
Carbohydrate	33 g
Fiber	1 g
Cholesterol	54 mg
Sodium	282 mg

Fettuccine Alfredo

* Large saucepan

1	package (12 oz/375 g) fresh fettuccine	1
½ cup	1% cottage cheese	125 mL
½ cup	1% milk	125 mL
⅓ cup	freshly grated Parmesan cheese	75 mL
Pinch	salt	Pinch
Pinch	freshly ground black pepper	Pinch
4 tsp	butter	20 mL
	Fresh snipped parsley (optional)	

1. In a large saucepan of boiling salted water, cook fettuccine for 3 minutes or according to package instructions, until tender to the bite. Drain and return to saucepan.

2. In a food processor or blender, process cottage cheese, milk, Parmesan, salt and pepper until smooth and creamy.

3. Over low heat, toss pasta with butter until melted. Stir in cottage cheese mixture, tossing gently, until pasta is uniformly coated and hot.

4. Sprinkle with fresh parsley, if using, and serve immediately.

Spaghetti and Meatballs (page 129) ▶
Overleaf: Picnic Hero (page 90)

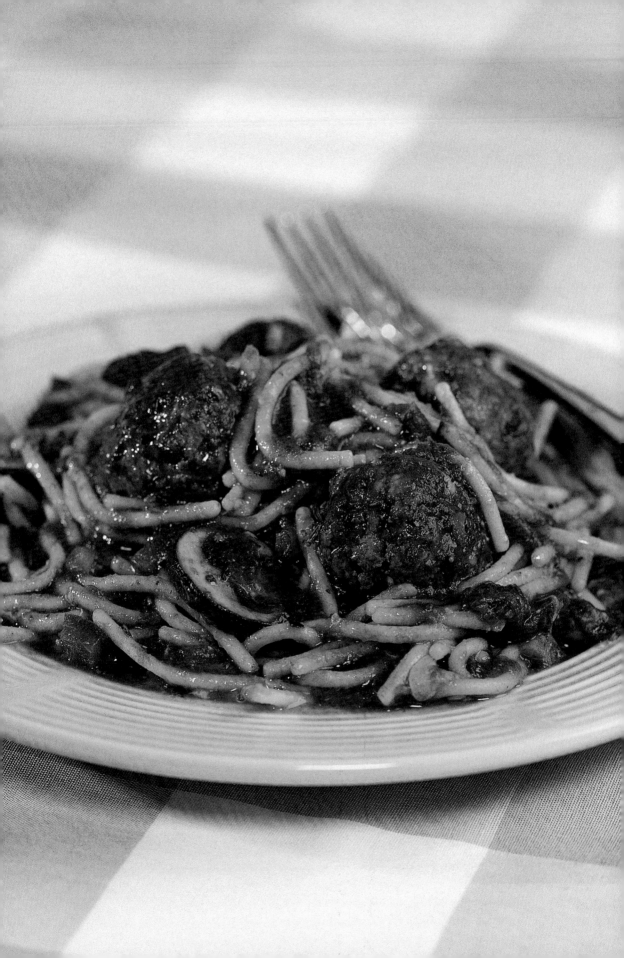

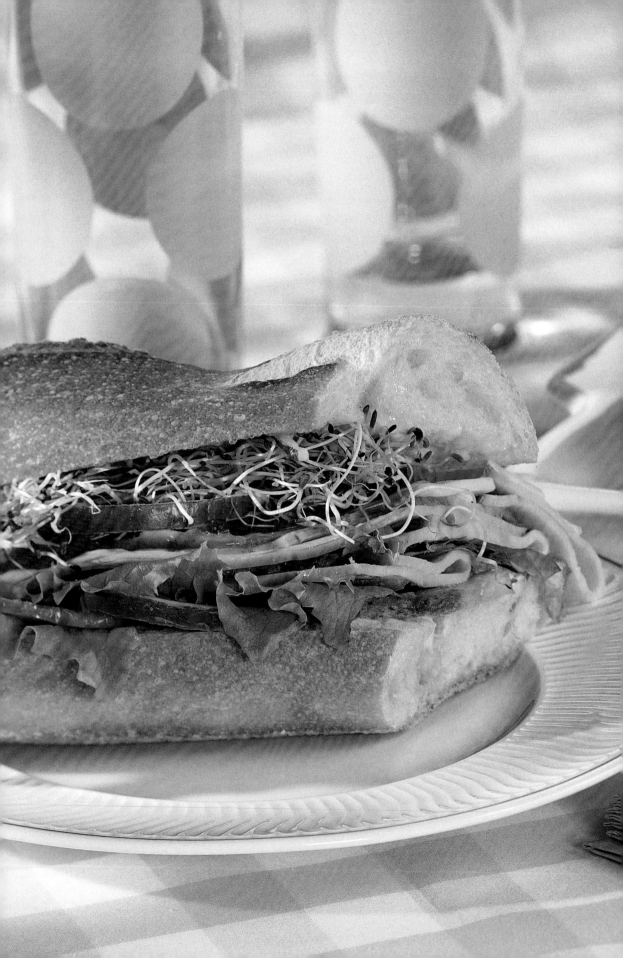

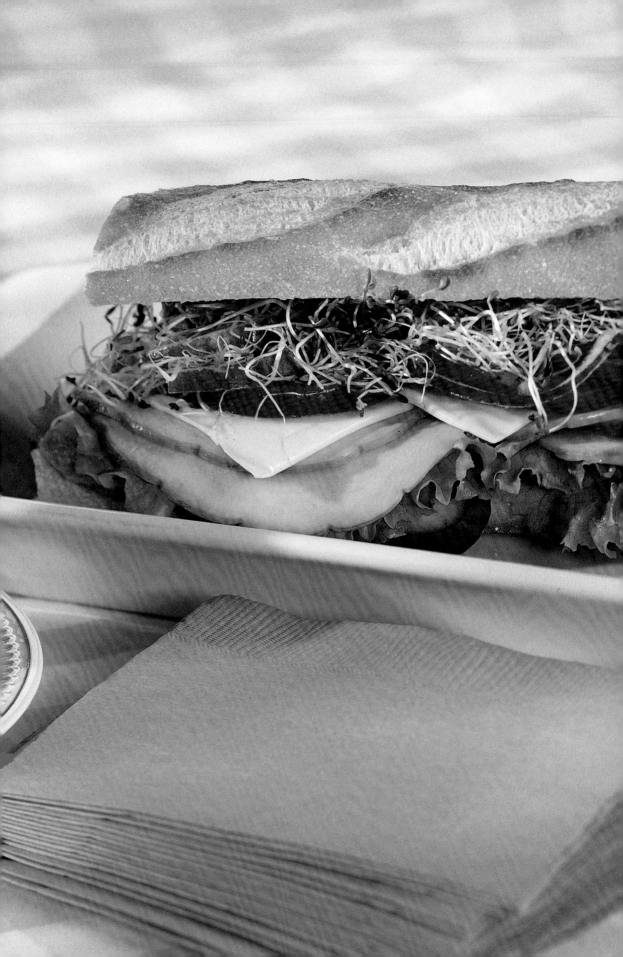

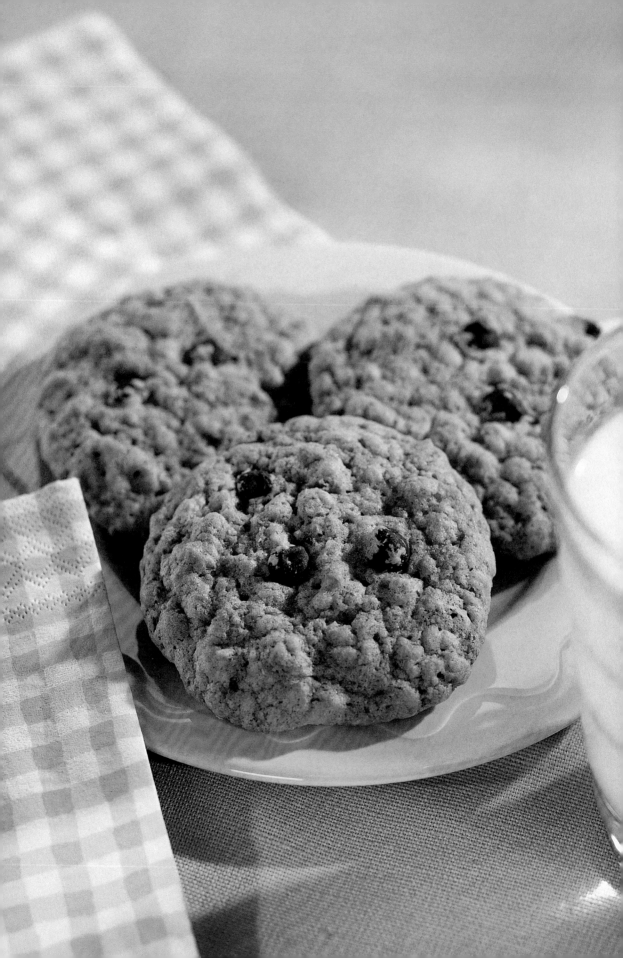

Spaghetti and Meatballs

I	large egg	I
12 oz	lean ground beef	375 g
2 tbsp	dry bread crumbs	25 mL
1½ tsp	salt, divided	7 mL
I	clove garlic, minced	I
½ cup	chopped onions	125 mL
I cup	sliced mushrooms	250 mL
½ cup	chopped green bell peppers	125 mL
I	can (19 oz/540 mL) diced tomatoes with juices	I
I tsp	dried Italian seasoning	5 mL
6 oz	spaghetti, broken into 2-inch (4 cm) pieces (about 1½ cups/375 mL)	175 g
I cup	shredded part-skim mozzarella cheese	250 mL

Prepare the meatballs ahead (see tip, below) or substitute frozen store-bought meatballs and make this easy one-pot dinner when you are camping.

Tip

To make meatballs in advance: Prepare the meatballs as in Step 1, but instead of frying them in a skillet, bake them on a baking sheet at 350°F (180°C) for 20 minutes, until cooked through. Cool completely. Cover and refrigerate for up to 2 days or freeze in an airtight container for up to 2 months.

1. In a medium bowl, combine egg, ground beef, bread crumbs and ½ tsp (2 mL) of the salt. Mix well and shape into 16 meatballs.

2. Heat a large, deep nonstick skillet, sprayed with vegetable spray, over medium-high heat. Cook the meatballs, turning often, for 5 to 6 minutes, until browned on all sides. Remove with a slotted spoon and set aside. Drain fat from skillet.

3. Reduce heat to medium and cook garlic and onions, stirring, for 2 minutes. Add mushrooms and green peppers and cook, stirring, for 3 to 4 minutes, until vegetables are tender. Return meatballs to the skillet.

4. Add tomatoes with juices, 1 cup (250 mL) water, spaghetti pieces, Italian seasoning and the remaining 1 tsp (5 mL) salt and bring to a boil. Reduce heat to medium-low, cover and simmer for 20 minutes, stirring occasionally, until pasta is tender and meatballs are no longer pink inside.

5. Sprinkle with mozzarella, stir until cheese is melted and serve.

◀ Chocolate Chip Cookies (page 138)

Exchanges Per Serving

2	Starch
3	Vegetable
3½	Lean Meat
2	Fat

Nutrient Analysis Per Serving

Calories	518
Protein	34 g
Fat	21 g
Saturated fat	9 g
Carbohydrate	49 g
Fiber	4 g
Cholesterol	121 mg
Sodium	1401 mg

Macaroni and cheese, a favorite comfort food, gets extra protein with the addition of canned salmon.

Tip

When using canned salmon, don't remove the bones, just mash them. They are an excellent source of calcium.

Salmon and Cheddar Macaroni

- *Preheat oven to 350°F (180°C)*
- *8-cup (2 L) baking dish, sprayed with vegetable spray*

I cup	macaroni	250 mL
4 tsp	soft margarine	20 mL
I	clove garlic, minced	I
¼ cup	finely chopped onions	50 mL
2 tbsp	all-purpose flour	25 mL
½ tsp	Worcestershire sauce	2 mL
I ½ cup	1% milk	375 mL
⅔ cup	shredded lower-fat Cheddar cheese, divided	150 mL
½ cup	lower-fat sour cream	125 mL
½ tsp	salt	2 mL
½ tsp	freshly ground black pepper	2 mL
I	can (7½ oz/213 g) sockeye salmon, drained	I
½ cup	dry bread crumbs	125 mL

1. Cook macaroni in 4 cups (1 L) boiling salted water according to package directions until tender to the bite. Drain carefully.

2. In a large saucepan, melt margarine over medium heat. Reserve 1 tsp (5 mL) of the margarine for later. Sauté garlic and onions for 3 minutes, or until onions are softened. Whisk in flour and cook, stirring, for 1 minute. Gradually whisk in milk and Worcestershire sauce, whisking until smooth. Continue to cook, whisking constantly, for 2 to 3 minutes, until mixture comes to a boil and thickens. Remove from heat.

3. Set aside 2 tbsp (25 mL) of the Cheddar. Add the rest to the sauce and stir until melted. Stir in sour cream, salt and pepper.

4. In a small bowl, flake salmon and mash bones with a fork, discarding skin; gently stir into the sauce. Stir in macaroni and transfer to prepared baking dish.

Exchanges Per Serving

2½ Starch

3 Lean Meat

I Fat

Nutrient Analysis Per Serving

Calories	434
Protein	29 g
Fat	16 g
Saturated fat	4 g
Carbohydrate	42 g
Fiber	2 g
Cholesterol	26 mg
Sodium	937 mg

5. In a small bowl, combine bread crumbs, reserved Cheddar and the reserved 1 tsp (5 mL) melted margarine. Sprinkle on top of macaroni.

6. Bake in preheated oven, uncovered, for 30 minutes, until topping is crisp and golden.

Dietitian's Message *Salmon contributes omega-3 fatty acids, which are hard to get without eating fatty fish. Other good sources include swordfish, mackerel, herring and sardines.*

These slightly sweet meatballs can be served as a main dish with rice, or as an appetizer. Or serve as hors d'oeuvres at a party, keeping them warm in a slow cooker.

Tip

To make 2 cups (500 mL) cooked rice:

Long-grain: Bring 1⅓ cups (325 mL) water to a boil; add ⅔ cup (150 mL) rice and ½ tsp (2 mL) salt. Stir, cover and simmer for 15 to 20 minutes, until water is absorbed. Fluff with a fork.

Exchanges Per Serving

1½	Starch
1	Fruit
½	Other Carbohydrate
2	Vegetable
2½	Lean Meat
2	Fat

Nutrient Analysis Per Serving

Calories	511
Protein	27 g
Fat	19 g
Saturated fat	7 g
Carbohydrate	58 g
Fiber	3 g
Cholesterol	118 mg
Sodium	942 mg

Sweet-and-Sour Meatballs

1	large egg	1
1 lb	lean ground beef	500 g
2 tbsp	dry bread crumbs	25 mL
½ tsp	salt	2 mL
2	carrots, sliced	2
1	onion, chopped	1
1	can (8 oz/227 mL) pineapple tidbits, with juices	1
3 tbsp	packed brown sugar	45 mL
2 tbsp	cornstarch	25 mL
3 tbsp	cider vinegar	45 mL
2 tbsp	soy sauce	25 mL
1 tbsp	ketchup	15 mL
½ cup	chopped green bell peppers	125 mL
2 cups	hot cooked rice	500 mL

1. In a medium bowl, combine egg, ground beef, bread crumbs and salt. Mix well and shape into 24 meatballs.

2. Heat a large nonstick skillet, sprayed with vegetable spray, over medium-high heat. Cook the meatballs, turning often, for 5 to 6 minutes, until browned on all sides. Remove meatballs with a slotted spoon and set aside. Drain fat from skillet.

3. Reduce heat to medium and stir-fry carrots and onion for 3 to 4 minutes, or until onion is softened.

4. Drain pineapple, reserving juice. Set pineapple aside.

5. In a small bowl, combine pineapple juice, brown sugar, vinegar, cornstarch, soy sauce and ketchup. Stir to dissolve the cornstarch. Add ½ cup (125 mL) water.

6. Pour juice mixture into the skillet with the carrots and onions. Cook, stirring constantly, for 2 to 3 minutes, until sauce thickens. Reduce heat to low.

7. Return meatballs to the skillet, cover and simmer for 15 minutes, until meatballs are no longer pink inside. Add pineapple and green peppers and cook for 5 minutes, until peppers are softened but still bright green.

8. Serve over hot rice.

Dietitian's Message *When buying ground beef, look for the description "lean" or "extra lean." Regular ground beef is high in fat, with over 15 grams per serving. One pound (500 g) of ground beef should feed four people.*

Brown rice: Bring 1¼ cups (300 mL) water to a boil; add ¾ cup (175 mL) rice and ½ tsp (2 mL) salt. Stir, cover and simmer for 35 to 40 minutes, until water is absorbed. Fluff with a fork.

Variations

Sweet-and-Sour Pork: Substitute 1 lb (500 g) pork tenderloin, cut into 1-inch (2.5 cm) cubes, for the meatball ingredients. Stir-fry pork cubes over medium-high heat for 5 to 6 minutes, until no longer pink inside. Remove from pan and proceed as above, starting with Step 3.

Sweet-and-Sour Chicken: Substitute 1 lb (500 g) skinless boneless chicken breasts or thighs, cut into chunks, for the meatball ingredients. Stir-fry chicken cubes over medium-high heat for 6 to 8 minutes, until no longer pink inside. Remove from pan and proceed as above, starting with Step 3.

Mini meatloaves take half the time to bake, and the individual servings make them more fun to eat.

Variation

You can makes these meatloaves spicier by adding hot pepper sauce and more chili powder. If you don't like spice, omit the chili powder and substitute ketchup for the salsa.

Exchanges Per Serving

1	Starch
3	Lean Meat
2	Fat

Nutrient Analysis Per Serving

Calories	280
Protein	22 g
Fat	14 g
Saturated fat	5 g
Carbohydrate	16 g
Fiber	2 g
Cholesterol	64 mg
Sodium	314 mg

Spicy Mini Meatloaves

- *Preheat oven to 350°F (180°C)*
- *12 nonstick muffin cups, sprayed with vegetable spray*

¼ cup	diced onions	50 mL
¼ cup	diced celery	50 mL
2	large eggs	2
12 oz	lean ground beef	375 g
8 oz	lean ground turkey	250 g
1½ cups	frozen corn kernels, thawed	375 mL
½ cup	quick-cooking rolled oats	125 mL
¼ cup	salsa	50 mL
1 tsp	chili powder	5 mL
½ tsp	salt	2 mL
½ tsp	freshly ground black pepper	2 mL

1. In a small microwave-safe bowl, mix onions and celery, cover with plastic wrap with one corner turned back, and microwave on High for 1 to 2 minutes, or until softened. Let cool.

2. In a large bowl, combine eggs, ground beef, ground turkey, corn, oats, salsa, chili powder, salt, pepper and the cooled vegetables. Shape into 12 portions and pack into prepared muffin cups.

3. Bake in preheated oven for 40 minutes, until meat is no longer pink inside and internal temperature has reached 170°F (75°C).

Dietitian's Message *The addition of cooked vegetables to burger and meatloaf recipes adds bulk, fiber and nutrients, and contributes to a moist texture.*

Saucy Pork Chops

- Preheat oven to 375°F (190°C)
- 13- by 9-inch (3 L) baking pan, sprayed with vegetable spray

4	bone-in pork loin chops (about 1 lb/500 g)	4
2	cloves garlic, minced	2
1/4 cup	salsa	50 mL
2 tbsp	ketchup	25 mL
1 tbsp	packed brown sugar	15 mL
1 tbsp	freshly squeezed lemon juice	15 mL
2 tsp	Worcestershire sauce	10 mL
1/2 tsp	salt	2 mL

1. Trim any visible fat from the pork chops and place in prepared pan.
2. In a small bowl, combine garlic, salsa, ketchup, brown sugar, lemon juice, Worcestershire sauce and salt. Spread evenly over pork chops.
3. Bake in preheated oven for 30 to 35 minutes, or until just a hint of pink remains in pork.

MAKES 4 SERVINGS

You can grill these chops on the barbecue if it is more convenient.

Variation

To grill the pork chops: Place chops in a shallow dish, pour in sauce and turn chops to coat evenly. Cover and refrigerate for at least 1 hour or overnight. Pour off sauce into a small saucepan and bring to a boil for at least 5 minutes. Set the saucepan on the barbecue and use the boiled sauce to baste the chops as they are grilling. Grill chops over medium heat for about 5 to 6 minutes per side, or until just a hint of pink remains in pork.

Exchanges Per Serving

1/2	Other Carbohydrate
3	Lean Meat

Nutrient Analysis Per Serving

Calories	158
Protein	21 g
Fat	5 g
Saturated fat	2 g
Carbohydrate	7 g
Fiber	0 g
Cholesterol	51 mg
Sodium	468 mg

Pork and fruit are a delicious combination. Make a pot of rice at the same time for a fast and easy dinner.

Tip

Meats with teriyaki-style sauces taste very good served with rice to soak up sauce. Try using an aromatic rice such as basmati or Texmati, which have a lovely nutty flavor and aroma.

Teriyaki Pork Chops with Apple Slices

- Preheat oven to 375°F (190°C)
- 13- by 9-inch (3 L) baking pan, sprayed with vegetable spray

4	bone-in pork loin chops (about 1 lb/500 g)	4
2 tbsp	soy sauce	25 mL
2 tsp	packed brown sugar	10 mL
1 tsp	Dijon mustard	5 mL
½ tsp	garlic powder	2 mL
½ tsp	ground ginger	2 mL
1	apple, cored and sliced, but not peeled	1

1. Trim any visible fat from the pork chops and place in prepared pan.
2. In a small bowl, combine soy sauce, brown sugar, Dijon mustard, garlic powder and ginger. Spread evenly over pork chops.
3. Bake in preheated oven for 20 minutes. Top pork chops with apple slices and continue to bake for 15 to 20 minutes, until just a hint of pink remains in pork.

Dietitian's Message *The apple in this recipe is a smart way to sneak in some fruit for the young one who shies away from fruits and vegetables. It sure makes the pork chops taste good too!*

Exchanges Per Serving

½ Other Carbohydrate

3 Lean Meat

Nutrient Analysis Per Serving

Calories	169
Protein	21 g
Fat	5 g
Saturated fat	2 g
Carbohydrate	9 g
Fiber	1 g
Cholesterol	51 mg
Sodium	546 mg

Baked Goodies

Chocolate Chip Cookies

Tip

Baking treats can hook kids on cooking. Encourage youngsters to bake by starting with an easy drop cookie such as this one. Baking, though, unlike cooking, is a science, and the ingredients must be measured exactly, so some supervision may be required.

Exchanges Per Serving

½	Starch
½	Other Carbohydrate
1	Fat

Nutrient Analysis Per Serving

Calories	145
Protein	2 g
Fat	7 g
Saturated fat	1 g
Carbohydrate	20 g
Fiber	1 g
Cholesterol	12 mg
Sodium	134 mg

- *Preheat oven to 350°F (180°C)*
- *Baking sheets, ungreased*

2 cups	all-purpose flour	500 mL
1 tsp	baking soda	5 mL
½ tsp	salt	2 mL
1 cup	soft margarine	250 mL
1 cup	granulated sugar	250 mL
½ cup	lightly packed brown sugar	125 mL
2	large eggs	2
2 tbsp	1% milk	25 mL
2 tsp	vanilla	10 mL
2⅓ cups	quick-cooking rolled oats	575 mL
½ cup	mini semi-sweet chocolate chips	125 mL

1. In a medium bowl, stir together flour, baking soda and salt.

2. In a large bowl, using an electric mixer or wooden spoon, beat margarine, granulated sugar and brown sugar until light and fluffy. Add eggs, milk and vanilla and beat well. Stir in flour mixture and mix well. Stir in oats and chocolate chips.

3. Drop by heaping tablespoonfuls (15 mL), about 2 inches (5 cm) apart, onto baking sheets. Bake in preheated oven for 16 to 18 minutes, or until slightly golden brown. Cool on baking sheets for 5 minutes, then remove to rack to cool completely.

Dietitian's Message *Rolled oats add texture to this classic cookie and contain soluble fiber, which will help slow the absorption of glucose from the chocolate chips and sugar. Serve with a tall glass of milk for an energizing snack.*

Peanut Butter Cookies

- Preheat oven to 350°F (180°C)
- Baking sheets, ungreased

1 cup	all-purpose flour	250 mL
½ tsp	salt	2 mL
½ tsp	baking soda	2 mL
½ cup	granulated sugar	125 mL
½ cup	lightly packed brown sugar	125 mL
⅓ cup	soft margarine	75 mL
1	large egg	1
⅔ cup	peanut butter	150 mL
½ tsp	vanilla	2 mL

1. In a small bowl, combine flour, salt and baking soda.

2. In a large bowl, using an electric mixer or wooden spoon, beat granulated sugar, brown sugar and margarine until light and fluffy. Beat in egg, peanut butter and vanilla. Stir in flour mixture until blended.

3. Roll dough into 36 small balls and place about 2 inches (5 cm) apart on baking sheets. Press flat with a floured fork. Bake in preheated oven for 10 to 12 minutes, or until lightly browned. Cool on baking sheets for 5 minutes, then remove to rack to cool completely.

Dietitian's Message *These crispy cookies are a good excuse for kids (and adults too!) to drink a glass of milk. Without enough milk, the daily quota of calcium and vitamin D is hard to get. The peanut butter packs a bit of protein as well.*

Tip

If you prefer to bake with artificial sweetener, your finished product will have a better texture if you substitute it for only some of the sugar. In this recipe, for example, substitute it for the granulated sugar. Also, add it with the dry ingredients instead of with the margarine.

**Exchanges
Per Serving**

½ Starch

½ Fat

**Nutrient Analysis
Per Serving**

Calories	80
Protein	2 g
Fat	4 g
Saturated fat	1 g
Carbohydrate	9 g
Fiber	0 g
Cholesterol	6 mg
Sodium	72 mg

Peanut butter chips add more yummy peanut flavor to these cookies, but you can substitute chocolate chips or make them with no chips at all.

Tip

For best results, keep your baking ingredients at room temperature. If your margarine or butter is cold, quickly soften it by placing it in a microwave-safe bowl and microwaving it, uncovered, for about 15 seconds on Medium-High (70%), just until it is softened but not melted.

**Exchanges
Per Serving**

$\frac{1}{2}$	Starch
1	Other Carbohydrate
$1\frac{1}{2}$	Fat

**Nutrient Analysis
Per Serving**

Calories	150
Protein	4 g
Fat	6 g
Saturated fat	2 g
Carbohydrate	21 g
Fiber	1 g
Cholesterol	11 mg
Sodium	153 mg

140

Peanut Butter Chip Cookies

- *Preheat oven to 350°F (180°C)*
- *Baking sheets, ungreased*

$1\frac{1}{2}$ cups	all-purpose flour	375 mL
$\frac{1}{2}$ cup	quick-cooking rolled oats	125 mL
$\frac{1}{2}$ tsp	salt	2 mL
$\frac{1}{2}$ tsp	baking soda	2 mL
$\frac{1}{2}$ cup	granulated sugar	125 mL
$\frac{1}{4}$ cup	lightly packed brown sugar	50 mL
$\frac{1}{4}$ cup	soft margarine	50 mL
1	large egg	1
1	large egg white	1
$\frac{1}{2}$ cup	lower-fat peanut butter	125 mL
$\frac{1}{2}$ tsp	vanilla	2 mL
$\frac{1}{2}$ cup	peanut butter chips	125 mL

1. In a medium bowl, stir together flour, oats, salt and baking soda.

2. In a large bowl, using an electric mixer or wooden spoon, beat granulated sugar, brown sugar and margarine until light and fluffy. Beat in egg, egg white, peanut butter and vanilla. Stir in flour mixture and mix well. Stir in peanut butter chips.

3. Roll into 40 small balls and place about 2 inches (5 cm) apart on baking sheets. Press flat with a floured fork. Bake in preheated oven for 8 to 10 minutes, or until lightly browned. Cool on baking sheets for 5 minutes, then remove to rack to cool completely.

Oatmeal Shortbread

- Baking sheets, ungreased

1 1/2 cups	all-purpose flour	375 mL
1 1/3 cups	quick-cooking rolled oats	325 mL
1 tsp	ground ginger	5 mL
1 tsp	salt	5 mL
3/4 cup	butter, softened	175 mL
1/4 cup	packed brown sugar	50 mL
1/4 cup	granulated sugar	50 mL
1/4 cup	unsweetened applesauce	50 mL
1 tsp	vanilla	5 mL

1. In a medium bowl, combine flour, oats, ginger and salt.

2. In a large bowl, using an electric mixer or wooden spoon, beat butter until creamy. Add brown sugar and granulated sugar and beat until light and fluffy. Stir in the applesauce and vanilla. Gradually stir in flour mixture until blended. Press the dough into a ball and knead slightly until smooth. Divide dough in half and shape each half into a roll about 2 inches (5 cm) in diameter. Wrap the rolls in waxed paper and refrigerate until firm, for at least 1 hour or overnight.

3. Preheat oven to 300°F (150°C). Cut chilled rolls of cookie dough into fifty 1/4-inch (0.5 cm) thick slices and place about 2 inches (5 cm) apart on baking sheets. Bake in preheated oven for 20 minutes, or until slightly golden brown. Cool on baking sheets for 5 minutes, then remove to rack to cool completely.

Dietitian's Message *Shortbread cookies are traditionally made with butter, which provides the characteristic rich, buttery flavor. If you wish, however, soft, non-hydrogenated tub margarine can be substituted.*

For Christmas, decorate these cookies with green and red sparkles or press half of a candied cherry on top of each.

Tip

Refrigerator cookie rolls can be wrapped in foil and refrigerated for up to 2 weeks or frozen in an airtight container for up to 2 months. When you are ready to bake, thaw the frozen rolls just until soft enough to slice.

Exchanges Per Serving

1/2	Starch
1/2	Other Carbohydrate
1	Fat

Nutrient Analysis Per Serving

Calories	116
Protein	2 g
Fat	6 g
Saturated fat	4 g
Carbohydrate	14 g
Fiber	1 g
Cholesterol	15 mg
Sodium	143 mg

Oatmeal Crunchies

Tip

Position the oven rack in the center of the oven when baking cookies. If you are baking 2 sheets at a time, switch the positions of the baking sheets halfway through baking.

Variations

Add ½ cup (125 mL) raisins, currants or chopped dates.

For a festive Christmas cookie, add ½ cup (125 mL) dried cranberries.

**Exchanges
Per Serving**

½	Starch
1	Other Carbohydrate
1½	Fat

**Nutrient Analysis
Per Serving**

Calories	136
Protein	2 g
Fat	6 g
Saturated fat	1 g
Carbohydrate	20 g
Fiber	1 g
Cholesterol	14 mg
Sodium	158 mg

- Preheat oven to 350°F (180°C)
- Baking sheets, ungreased

1 cup	all-purpose flour	250 mL
1 tsp	salt	5 mL
½ tsp	baking soda	2 mL
1 cup	lightly packed brown sugar	250 mL
½ cup	granulated sugar	125 mL
¾ cup	soft margarine	175 mL
2	large eggs	2
1 tsp	vanilla	5 mL
2⅔ cups	quick-cooking rolled oats	650 mL

1. In a small bowl, combine flour, salt and baking soda.

2. In a large bowl, using an electric mixer or wooden spoon, beat brown sugar, granulated sugar and margarine until light and fluffy. Add eggs and vanilla and beat until smooth. Gradually stir in flour mixture and mix well. Stir in oats.

3. Drop by heaping tablespoonfuls (15 mL), about 2 inches (5 cm) apart, onto baking sheets. Bake in preheated oven for 12 to 15 minutes, or until golden brown. Cool on baking sheets for 5 minutes, then remove to rack to cool completely.

Dietitian's Message *These cookies have a good portion of rolled oats, which are rich in soluble fiber. Soluble fiber lowers blood cholesterol, as well as the glycemic index of the cookies.*

Applesauce Spice Cookies

A moist and delicious old-fashioned cookie!

- Preheat oven to 350°F (180°C)
- Baking sheets, ungreased

1 ¼ cups	all-purpose flour	300 mL
1 tsp	baking powder	5 mL
1 tsp	pumpkin pie spice	5 mL
½ tsp	baking soda	2 mL
¼ tsp	salt	1 mL
¾ cup	soft margarine	175 mL
½ cup	granulated sugar	125 mL
¼ cup	lightly packed brown sugar	50 mL
1	large egg	1
½ tsp	vanilla	2 mL
1 cup	unsweetened applesauce	250 mL
1 ⅓ cups	quick-cooking rolled oats	325 mL
½ cup	currants or raisins	125 mL

1. In a medium bowl, stir together flour, baking powder, pumpkin pie spice, baking soda and salt.

2. In a large bowl, beat margarine, granulated sugar and brown sugar until light and fluffy. Add egg and vanilla and beat well.

3. Gradually stir in flour mixture alternately with applesauce, making 3 or 4 additions of each, and mix well. Stir in rolled oats and currants.

4. Drop by heaping tablespoonfuls (15 mL), about 2 inches (5 cm) apart, onto baking sheets. Bake in preheated oven for 12 to 15 minutes, or until lightly browned. Cool on baking sheets for 5 minutes, then remove to rack to cool completely.

Dietitian's Message *The currants or raisins help to naturally sweeten these flavorful cookies. Paired with yogurt, they make a tasty after-school snack.*

Tips

Out of pumpkin pie spice? Substitute ¾ tsp (4 mL) ground cinnamon and ¼ tsp (1 mL) ground nutmeg or ginger.

These cookies have a muffin-like texture and get softer after storing at room temperature. If you plan to store them for more than 2 days, place them in an airtight container and freeze.

Exchanges Per Serving

½	Starch
½	Other Carbohydrate
1½	Fat

Nutrient Analysis Per Serving

Calories	156
Protein	2 g
Fat	8 g
Saturated fat	1 g
Carbohydrate	20 g
Fiber	1 g
Cholesterol	11 mg
Sodium	162 mg

Meringue Candy Canes

The secret to perfect meringues is to bake them at a low temperature in the center of the oven for a long time.

- *Preheat oven to 200°F (100°C)*
- *2 baking sheets, lined with parchment paper*
- *Large pastry bag with ½-inch (1 cm) plain tip*
- *Medium pastry bag with ¼-inch (0.5 cm) plain tip*

Tips

Eggs separate more easily when cold, but egg whites gain more volume when beaten at room temperature. To warm to room temperature, place bowl of egg whites in a larger bowl of hot water and let stand for 5 minutes.

For best results when making meringues, use a clean stainless steel or glass bowl to beat the egg whites.

4	large egg whites, at room temperature	4
½ tsp	cream of tartar	2 mL
¼ tsp	salt	1 mL
⅔ cup	granulated sugar	150 mL
½ tsp	peppermint extract	2 mL
	Red food coloring	

1. Using a pencil, lightly draw 48 candy cane shapes on the parchment paper; flip the paper over.

2. Position oven racks in the center of the oven.

3. In a large bowl, using an electric mixer, beat egg whites, cream of tartar and salt at medium speed until foamy. Continue beating, adding sugar 2 tbsp (25 mL) at a time, until stiff, glossy peaks form, then beat in peppermint extract. Transfer ½ cup (125 mL) to a small bowl and stir in a few drops of red food coloring to tint pink.

4. Fill the large pastry bag with the white meringue and pipe onto the candy cane shapes on the parchment paper. Fill the medium pastry bag with the pink meringue and pipe into diagonal stripes across the candy canes.

5. Bake in preheated oven for 1¼ hours until firm. Turn heat off and leave meringues to dry in oven for 1 hour. Peel meringues off parchment paper and transfer to a rack to cool completely.

Exchanges
Per Serving

½ Other Carbohydrate

Nutrient Analysis
Per Serving

Calories	25
Protein	1 g
Fat	0 g
Saturated fat	0 g
Carbohydrate	6 g
Fiber	0 g
Cholesterol	0 mg
Sodium	32 mg

Christmas Brownies

- Preheat oven to 300°F (150°C)
- 9-inch (2.5 L) square baking pan, sprayed with vegetable spray

The colorful topping makes these brownies an attractive addition to a Christmas cookie tray.

24	lower-fat graham wafers	24
2 tbsp	unsweetened cocoa powder	25 mL
1/2 tsp	salt	2 mL
2	large eggs	2
1	large egg white	1
1/3 cup	packed brown sugar	75 mL
1/4 cup	granulated sugar	50 mL
2 tsp	vanilla	10 mL
1/2 cup	white chocolate chips	125 mL
1/2 cup	slivered almonds	125 mL
1/3 cup	coarsely chopped dried cranberries	75 mL

Tip

Because it is easy to overcook the base, always bake bars in the center of the oven and check for doneness at the minimum suggested baking time.

1. In a food processor, pulse wafers into coarse crumbs. (Or place wafers on a large sheet of waxed paper, cover with another sheet of waxed paper and crush with a rolling pin.) Add cocoa and salt and process until combined.

2. In a large bowl, using an electric mixer or wooden spoon, beat eggs, egg white, brown sugar, granulated sugar and vanilla until well blended and thickened. Stir in crumb mixture.

3. Spread batter evenly in prepared pan and sprinkle with chocolate chips, almonds and cranberries. Press toppings gently into the batter so they will adhere when baked.

4. Bake in preheated oven for 25 to 30 minutes, or until knife inserted in the center comes out clean. Let cool completely in pan on a rack and cut into 16 squares.

Exchanges Per Serving

1	Other Carbohydrate
1	Fat

Nutrient Analysis Per Serving

Calories	124
Protein	2 g
Fat	6 g
Saturated fat	2 g
Carbohydrate	18 g
Fiber	1 g
Cholesterol	27 mg
Sodium	24 mg

Chocolate Brownies

Tip

Unsweetened cocoa powder has only 115 calories and 4 grams of fat per ⅓ cup (75 mL), whereas 1 oz (25 g) of unsweetened baking chocolate has 139 calories and 14 grams of fat. Cocoa has just as much rich chocolate flavor as baking chocolate, so substituting cocoa is a good way to cut fat.

- Preheat oven to 350°F (180°C)
- 8-inch (2 L) square baking pan, sprayed with vegetable spray

⅔ cup	all-purpose flour	150 mL
½ cup	granulated sugar	125 mL
⅓ cup	unsweetened cocoa powder, sifted	75 mL
1 tsp	baking powder	5 mL
¼ tsp	salt	1 mL
⅓ cup	chopped walnuts	75 mL
2	large eggs	2
⅓ cup	soft margarine	75 mL
1 tsp	vanilla	5 mL
½ cup	unsweetened applesauce	125 mL

1. In a medium bowl, stir together flour, sugar, cocoa, baking powder and salt. Stir in walnuts.

2. In a small bowl, using an electric mixer, beat eggs, margarine and vanilla at high speed for 1 minute, until well mixed. Add applesauce and beat just until blended. Add flour mixture and mix at low speed just until blended.

3. Spread batter evenly in prepared pan and bake in preheated oven for 15 minutes, until a knife inserted in the center comes out clean. Let cool completely in pan on a rack and cut into 16 squares.

Exchanges Per Serving

½ Starch

½ Other Carbohydrate

1 Fat

Nutrient Analysis Per Serving

Calories	111
Protein	2 g
Fat	6 g
Saturated fat	1 g
Carbohydrate	13 g
Fiber	1 g
Cholesterol	27 mg
Sodium	106 mg

Crispy Granola Squares

- 13- by 9-inch (3 L) baking pan, lined with foil and sprayed with vegetable spray

¼ cup	soft margarine	50 mL
3 cups	mini marshmallows	750 mL
5 cups	crisp rice cereal	1.25 L
¼ cup	unsweetened cocoa powder, sifted	50 mL
1 tsp	vanilla	5 mL
⅓ cup	quick-cooking rolled oats	75 mL
⅓ cup	unsweetened flaked coconut	75 mL
¼ cup	raisins	50 mL
¼ cup	semi-sweet chocolate chips	50 mL

These crispy squares are fun for kids to make, but be careful to mix quickly and thoroughly once you have added all the ingredients to the melted marshmallows.

Tips

So you can get the squares out of the pan easily, allow the foil to extend over the edges of the pan.

To cut easily into neat squares, dip your knife in hot water before each cut.

1. In a large, heavy saucepan, over low heat, melt margarine. Add marshmallows and stir constantly until marshmallows are melted, about 10 minutes. Remove from heat, stir in rice cereal, cocoa and vanilla and mix until evenly coated. Add oats, coconut, raisins and chocolate chips and mix until evenly coated.

2. Press evenly into prepared baking pan. Refrigerate for 30 minutes to 1 hour, until firm. Using foil, lift the bars out of the pan and cut into 24 squares.

Dietitian's Message *Crisp rice cereal is fortified with B vitamins, and the carbohydrate from the marshmallows, raisins and chocolate chips can be readily be fit into the meal plan of active children. School-age kids will love finding these squares as a surprise in their lunch.*

**Exchanges
Per Serving**

1	Other Carbohydrate
1	Fat

**Nutrient Analysis
Per Serving**

Calories	94
Protein	1 g
Fat	4 g
Saturated fat	2 g
Carbohydrate	15 g
Fiber	1 g
Cholesterol	0 mg
Sodium	84 mg

This moist and easy tropical cake should be stored in the refrigerator. It will keep for 2 to 3 days.

Piña Colada Snacking Cake

- Preheat oven to 350°F (180°C)
- 13- by 9-inch (3 L) baking pan, sprayed with vegetable spray

2 cups	all-purpose flour	500 mL
1/2 cup	packed brown sugar	125 mL
1/2 cup	shredded unsweetened coconut	125 mL
1 tsp	ground cinnamon	5 mL
1/2 tsp	ground ginger	2 mL
1/2 tsp	salt	2 mL
2	large eggs	2
1	can (19 oz/540 mL) crushed pineapple, in juice	1
1/4 cup	confectioner's (icing) sugar, sifted	50 mL

1. In a large bowl, combine flour, brown sugar, coconut, cinnamon, ginger and salt.

2. In a small bowl, mix eggs well with a fork. Add pineapple and juice and stir to combine. Add to flour mixture and stir until blended.

3. Pour batter into prepared pan and bake in preheated oven for 25 to 30 minutes, or until a knife inserted in the center comes out clean. Let cool completely in pan on a rack and cut into 16 squares.

4. In a small bowl, mix confectioner's sugar with about 1 tbsp (15 mL) water to make a thin glaze. Transfer to an icing bag and drizzle onto cooled squares.

Dietitian's Message *Kids can easily prepare this recipe with a little supervision — and there's little cleanup involved. Supervise the portioning, though, as the cake tastes great!*

Exchanges Per Serving

1	Starch
1/2	Other Carbohydrate

Nutrient Analysis Per Serving

Calories	136
Protein	3 g
Fat	2 g
Saturated fat	2 g
Carbohydrate	27 g
Fiber	1 g
Cholesterol	27 mg
Sodium	80 mg

Chocolate Banana Muffins

Hearty, nutritious muffins are great any time of day for families on the go.

- Preheat oven to 425°F (220°C)
- 12 muffin cups, lined with paper liners or sprayed with vegetable spray

2 cups	all-purpose flour	500 mL
²⁄₃ cup	natural bran	150 mL
¹⁄₄ cup	unsweetened cocoa powder, sifted	50 mL
1 tsp	baking powder	5 mL
1 tsp	baking soda	5 mL
1 tsp	salt	5 mL
1	large egg	1
1	large egg white	1
1 cup	buttermilk	250 mL
¹⁄₄ cup	vegetable oil	50 mL
1 tsp	vanilla	5 mL
2	medium bananas, mashed (about 1 cup/250 mL)	2
¹⁄₃ cup	packed brown sugar	75 mL
¹⁄₂ cup	peanut butter chips	125 mL

1. In a large bowl, combine flour, bran, cocoa, baking powder, baking soda and salt.

2. In a medium bowl, whisk together egg, egg white, buttermilk, oil and vanilla until well blended. Stir in bananas and brown sugar. Make a well in the center of the dry ingredients, pour in the egg mixture and stir just until blended. Stir in peanut butter chips.

3. Spoon batter into prepared muffin cups and bake in preheated oven for 15 to 17 minutes, or until firm. Let cool in pan on a rack for 10 minutes. Transfer to a rack to cool completely.

Tip

If you like a crispier crust on your muffins, grease the muffin tins (or spray with vegetable spray) instead of using paper liners. Grease the bottoms of the tins only — greasing the sides stops the tops from rounding as nicely.

Exchanges Per Serving

1	Starch
¹⁄₂	Fruit
1	Other Carbohydrate
2	Fat

Nutrient Analysis Per Serving

Calories	249
Protein	5 g
Fat	10 g
Saturated fat	3 g
Carbohydrate	39 g
Fiber	4 g
Cholesterol	19 mg
Sodium	337 mg

Peanut Butter Muffins

Don't let the long list of ingredients scare you. These muffins are so tasty and filling that they are worth the effort.

Tips
You will need a 12-cup muffin pan and a 6-cup muffin pan.

For fresh muffins in the morning, mix dry ingredients and liquid ingredients in 2 separate containers and store in the refrigerator overnight. In the morning, stir the liquid ingredients into the dry ingredients and bake, adding 5 to 10 minutes to the baking time.

Exchanges Per Serving

1	Starch
½	Other Carbohydrate
1	High-Fat Meat
1	Fat

Nutrient Analysis Per Serving

Calories	210
Protein	7 g
Fat	10 g
Saturated fat	3 g
Carbohydrate	25 g
Fiber	3 g
Cholesterol	36 mg
Sodium	273 mg

- Preheat oven to 375°F (190°C)
- 18 muffin cups, lined with paper liners or sprayed with vegetable spray

1½ cups	whole wheat flour	375 mL
1¼ cups	quick-cooking rolled oats	300 mL
½ cup	granulated sugar	125 mL
¼ cup	wheat germ	50 mL
4 tsp	baking powder	20 mL
1 tsp	baking soda	5 mL
1 tsp	salt	5 mL
⅓ cup	mini semi-sweet chocolate chips	75 mL
3	large eggs	3
1 cup	plain yogurt	250 mL
½ cup	buttermilk	125 mL
½ cup	peanut butter	125 mL
¼ cup	vegetable oil	50 mL
1 tsp	vanilla	5 mL

1. In a large bowl, combine flour, oats, sugar, wheat germ, baking powder, baking soda and salt. Stir in chocolate chips.

2. In a medium bowl, whisk together eggs, yogurt, buttermilk, peanut butter, oil and vanilla until smooth and well blended. Pour into flour mixture and stir just until blended.

3. Spoon batter into prepared muffin cups and bake in preheated oven for 20 to 25 minutes, or until firm. Let cool in pan on a rack for 10 minutes. Transfer to a rack to cool completely.

Dietitian's Message *Whole wheat flour and rolled oats contribute fiber, which is indigestible and traps carbohydrate on its way through the digestive system. The more fiber content in a recipe, the less total carbohydrate will be available to affect blood sugars.*

Potato Cheese Muffins

- Preheat oven to 400°F (200°C)
- 10 muffin cups, lined with paper cups or sprayed with vegetable spray

2 cups	all-purpose flour	500 mL
1/3 cup	granulated sugar	75 mL
4 tsp	baking powder	20 mL
1 tsp	salt	5 mL
2	large eggs	2
1 1/2 cups	1% milk	375 mL
3/4 cup	shredded lower-fat Cheddar cheese	175 mL
1/2 cup	mashed cooked potato (about 1 potato)	125 mL
1/3 cup	soft margarine, melted	75 mL

1. In a large bowl, combine flour, granulated sugar, baking powder and salt.

2. In a medium bowl, using an electric mixer or a wooden spoon, beat eggs well. Stir in milk, cheese, mashed potato and margarine and mix well. Add to flour mixture and stir just until blended.

3. Spoon batter into prepared muffin tins and bake in preheated oven for 25 minutes, or until firm and lightly browned. Let cool in pan on a rack for 10 minutes. Transfer to a rack. Best served warm from the oven.

Dietitian's Message *This savory muffin is perfect for lunch. Pack a low-sugar yogurt and an orange for additional protein, calcium and vitamin C.*

Serve these freshly baked muffins for breakfast or with a bowl of soup or chili on a frosty winter's day.

Tip

Over-mixing muffin batter will make muffins tough, flat-topped and full of tunnels. The rule of thumb is to stir gently just until the wet and dry ingredients are combined.

Exchanges Per Serving

1 1/2	Starch
1/2	Other Carbohydrate
1	High-Fat Meat
1	Fat

Nutrient Analysis Per Serving

Calories	290
Protein	10 g
Fat	14 g
Saturated fat	5 g
Carbohydrate	31 g
Fiber	1 g
Cholesterol	64 mg
Sodium	537 mg

Banana bread is good for a quick breakfast, dessert or afternoon tea.

Tip

Don't compost your overripe bananas — turn them into banana bread! The riper the bananas, the sweeter the bread. This bread tastes best the day after you bake it.

Exchanges Per Serving

1	Starch
1/2	Fruit
1	Other Carbohydrate
2	Fat

Nutrient Analysis Per Serving

Calories	276
Protein	5 g
Fat	11 g
Saturated fat	1 g
Carbohydrate	42 g
Fiber	2 g
Cholesterol	43 mg
Sodium	269 mg

Banana Bread

- Preheat oven to 350°F (180°C)
- 9- by 5-inch (2 L) loaf pan, sprayed with vegetable spray and dusted with flour

2 cups	all-purpose flour	500 mL
1 tsp	baking powder	5 mL
1 tsp	baking soda	5 mL
1/2 tsp	salt	2 mL
2	large eggs	2
1 cup	mashed ripe bananas (about 2 medium)	250 mL
1/2 cup	chopped walnuts	125 mL
1/2 cup	granulated sugar	125 mL
1/4 cup	lightly packed brown sugar	50 mL
1/4 cup	vegetable oil	50 mL
1/4 cup	unsweetened applesauce	50 mL

1. In a medium bowl, mix together flour, baking powder, baking soda and salt.

2. In a large bowl, using an electric mixer or a wooden spoon, beat eggs, bananas, walnuts, granulated sugar, brown sugar, oil and applesauce until well mixed. Stir in flour mixture just until blended.

3. Pour batter into prepared loaf pan and bake in preheated oven for 55 to 60 minutes, or until a knife inserted in the center comes out clean. Cool in the pan on a rack for 15 minutes. Remove from pan and let cool completely on a rack.

Dietitian's Message *Bananas contain soluble fiber and lots of potassium. Very ripe bananas work best in this recipe because they are the easiest to mash. If you have extra bananas, you can mash and then freeze them in an airtight container for up to 1 month.*

Desserts

Strawberry Delights

Celebrate strawberry season with this fun-to-make recipe that kids can prepare on their own!

Tip

On your next picnic, take along fresh strawberries, cream cheese mixture and sprinkles in separate containers. Arrange strawberries on a platter surrounding the toppings and let everyone dip berries in the cream cheese mixture and the sprinkles.

24	large strawberries	24
4 oz	lower-fat cream cheese, at room temperature	125 g
2 tbsp	granulated sugar	25 mL
1 1/2 tsp	freshly squeezed lemon juice	7 mL
1/4 cup	chocolate sprinkles	50 mL

1. Wash strawberries and pat dry with a paper towel.

2. In a small bowl, combine cream cheese, sugar and lemon juice. Blend well.

3. Holding each strawberry by its leaf, dip the bottom half of the strawberry into the cream cheese mixture, coating it well. Then dip it in chocolate sprinkles and set on waxed paper.

4. Repeat until all strawberries are dipped. Arrange on a serving plate and serve immediately or cover and refrigerate for up to 2 hours.

Dietitian's Message *It's all in the presentation! This is such a scrumptious little treat, and it's quite simple to make. The strawberries are a source of vitamin C and fiber, while the cream cheese and chocolate sprinkles add only 3 grams of fat.*

Exchanges Per Serving

1/2	Other Carbohydrate
1/2	Fat

Nutrient Analysis Per Serving

Calories	62
Protein	1 g
Fat	3 g
Saturated fat	2 g
Carbohydrate	8 g
Fiber	1 g
Cholesterol	7 mg
Sodium	75 mg

Fruit on a Cloud

A very pretty way to serve fresh fruit!

- *Baking sheet, lined with waxed paper*

4 oz	lower-fat cream cheese	125 g
1 cup	lower-fat non-dairy whipped topping	250 mL
1 cup	miniature marshmallows	250 mL
2 cups	mixed fresh fruit, such as raspberries, blueberries, grapes, and sliced nectarines	500 mL

1. In a medium bowl, using an electric mixer, beat cream cheese until light and fluffy. Add whipped topping, adjust mixer to slow setting and stir until smooth, about 2 minutes. Stir in marshmallows.

2. To make clouds, spoon cream cheese mixture in 4 mounds onto prepared baking sheet. Spread each mound into a 3-inch (7.5 cm) circle with the back of a spoon and make a deep well in the center of each circle, building up the sides. Freeze for 2 to 3 hours.

3. Remove clouds from the freezer and place on individual serving plates. Let stand at room temperature for 15 minutes.

4. Meanwhile, combine fruit in a small bowl.

5. Spoon 1/2 cup (125 mL) fruit into the center of each cloud and serve immediately.

Dietitian's Message *This dessert is high in carbohydrates because of the marshmallows, but it can be a good way to encourage a child who avoids eating fruit to eat some. Fruits are good sources of vitamin C, beta carotene, antioxidants and fiber.*

Tip
Use your favorite fruit and berries.

Variation
Drizzle calorie-reduced sundae topping over the fruit. Or garnish with fresh sliced strawberries and drizzle with Chocolate Sauce (see recipe, page 159).

Exchanges Per Serving

1/2	Fruit
1	Other Carbohydrate
1/2	Medium-Fat Meat
1/2	Fat

Nutrient Analysis Per Serving

Calories	151
Protein	3 g
Fat	5 g
Saturated fat	3 g
Carbohydrate	25 g
Fiber	2 g
Cholesterol	18 mg
Sodium	168 mg

The addition of mini marshmallows and yogurt changes an ordinary fruit salad into a special dessert.

Creamy Dreamy Fruit Salad

1	apple, cored and diced	1
2 tsp	freshly squeezed lemon juice	10 mL
1	can (14 oz/398 mL) pineapple tidbits, packed in juice, drained	1
1	can (10 oz/284 mL) mandarin orange sections, drained	1
1 cup	halved seedless grapes	250 mL
1 cup	mini marshmallows	250 mL
¾ cup	1% or 2% orange- or pineapple-flavored yogurt	175 mL
2	medium bananas	2

1. In a large bowl, toss diced apple with lemon juice to prevent browning. Add pineapple, mandarin oranges, grapes and marshmallows.

2. Drizzle with yogurt and toss gently until fruit and marshmallows are evenly coated. Refrigerate for at least 1 hour or for up to 8 hours to blend flavors.

3. Just before serving, slice bananas and stir into fruit mixture.

Dietitian's Message *This mix of fruit and yogurt makes a tasty, nutritious dessert. It can be a light finish to a heartier meal. Try teaming it with Oven-Baked Crispy Chicken (see recipe, page 113).*

Exchanges Per Serving

2   Fruit

Nutrient Analysis Per Serving

Calories	128
Protein	2 g
Fat	1 g
Saturated fat	0 g
Carbohydrate	31 g
Fiber	1 g
Cholesterol	2 mg
Sodium	18 mg

Quick Chocolate Mousse

This easy mousse can be enjoyed as it is, or can be used to make other desserts, such as Ice Cream Fantasy Cake (see recipe, page 162).

1	package (1½ oz/40 g) fat-free instant chocolate pudding mix, sweetened with aspartame	1
1½ cups	cold 1% milk	375 mL
2 cups	lower-fat non-dairy whipped topping	500 mL

1. In a medium bowl, add chocolate pudding mix to milk. Beat for 1 minute, then fold in whipped topping. Let stand for 5 minutes to set; serve immediately or cover with waxed paper and refrigerate overnight.

Exchanges Per Serving

1½ Low-Fat Milk

½ Other Carbohydrate

Nutrient Analysis Per Serving

Calories	84
Protein	3 g
Fat	2 g
Saturated fat	1 g
Carbohydrate	14 g
Fiber	0 g
Cholesterol	9 mg
Sodium	124 mg

No-sugar-added pudding mixes and a little imagination can be the basis for easy, quick desserts.

Rocky Road Mousse

1	package (1½ oz/40 g) fat-free instant chocolate pudding mix, sweetened with aspartame	1
1½ cups	cold 1% milk	375 mL
1 cup	lower-fat non-dairy whipped topping	250 mL
½ cup	plain yogurt	125 mL
6	lower-fat graham wafers	6
1 cup	miniature marshmallows	250 ml
½ cup	Chocolate Sauce (see recipe, facing page)	125 mL

1. In a medium bowl, add chocolate pudding mix to milk. Beat for 1 minute, then fold in whipped topping and yogurt. Divide among 6 dessert dishes or parfait glasses. Let stand for 5 minutes until set, or cover and refrigerate for up to 4 hours.

2. Just before serving, break graham wafers into small pieces and sprinkle one wafer on each mousse. Top with mini marshmallows and drizzle with chocolate sauce.

Exchanges Per Serving

½ Starch

1 Other Carbohydrate

½ Medium-Fat Meat

Nutrient Analysis Per Serving

Calories	130
Protein	4 g
Fat	2 g
Saturated fat	1 g
Carbohydrate	24 g
Fiber	0 g
Cholesterol	6 mg
Sodium	176 mg

Chocolate Sauce

¼ cup	unsweetened cocoa powder, sifted	50 mL
1 tbsp	cornstarch	15 mL
¾ cup	evaporated skim milk	175 mL
½ cup	granulated sugar	125 mL
1 tsp	vanilla	5 mL

**MAKES
1 CUP (250 ML)
or 8 servings
(2 tbsp/25 mL
per serving)**

This sauce can be stored in the fridge for up to 3 days and used as a topping for many desserts.

1. In a small saucepan, combine cocoa and cornstarch. Whisk in ¼ cup (50 mL) of water until smooth. Whisk in milk and cook over low heat, stirring constantly, until the mixture comes to a boil, about 5 minutes. Cook for 1 minute longer, stirring constantly, until thickened (it will thicken more as it cools).

2. Remove from heat and stir in sugar and vanilla. Let cool to room temperature. Cover and refrigerate for up to 3 days.

Dietitian's Message *This sauce is delicious over vanilla ice cream or fresh strawberries. If the carbohydrate content is higher than you would like, replace sugar with an amount of artificial sweetener that has the same amount of sweetening power as ½ cup (125 mL) sugar. Using artificial sweetener will reduce the calories to 37 and the carbohydrate content to 7 g/serving.*

**Exchanges
Per Serving**

1	Other Carbohydrate

**Nutrient Analysis
Per Serving**

Calories	85
Protein	2 g
Fat	0 g
Saturated fat	0 g
Carbohydrate	18 g
Fiber	1 g
Cholesterol	1 mg
Sodium	27 mg

This dessert is easy to make, and the look and taste are elegant!

Variation

Maple Walnut and Pear Tiramisu: Substitute vanilla pudding for the chocolate pudding and a 14-oz (398 mL) can of pear halves (packed in pear juice) for the bananas. Add ¼ cup (50 mL) chopped walnuts to the middle layer. Do not put pears in the middle layer, but add ¼ cup (50 mL) pear juice to the pudding mixture. Garnish the top of the tiramisu with the pear halves down the middle.

Exchanges Per Serving

1	Starch
½	Other Carbohydrate
1	Fat

Nutrient Analysis Per Serving

Calories	150
Protein	4 g
Fat	5 g
Saturated fat	1 g
Carbohydrate	24 g
Fiber	1 g
Cholesterol	64 mg
Sodium	48 mg

Banana Cream Tiramisu

- 9- by 5-inch (2 L) loaf pan, lined with waxed paper

12	giant ladyfinger biscuits (about 5 oz/150 g)	12
3 tbsp	pure maple syrup, divided	45 mL
1 cup	lower-fat non-dairy whipped topping	250 mL
1 cup	prepared fat-free chocolate pudding, made with 1% milk	250 mL
1	large banana	1
¼ cup	chopped walnuts	50 mL

1. Arrange 6 ladyfingers in a single layer across the bottom of prepared loaf pan. Drizzle evenly with 2 tbsp (25 mL) of the maple syrup.

2. In a medium bowl, fold whipped topping into chocolate pudding.

3. Slice ⅔ banana and arrange in single layer over the ladyfingers. Spoon ½ of the pudding mixture over the banana and spread evenly. Wrap the remaining banana and set aside.

4. Arrange the remaining 6 ladyfingers in single layer over the pudding and drizzle the remaining 1 tbsp (15 mL) maple syrup over the ladyfingers. Dollop (or pipe) the rest of the pudding mixture onto the ladyfingers. Cover and refrigerate for at least 1 hour or for up to 1 day.

5. Just before serving, slice the remaining banana and arrange decoratively down the center of the tiramisu. Sprinkle with chopped walnuts.

Crispy Granola Squares (page 147) ▶

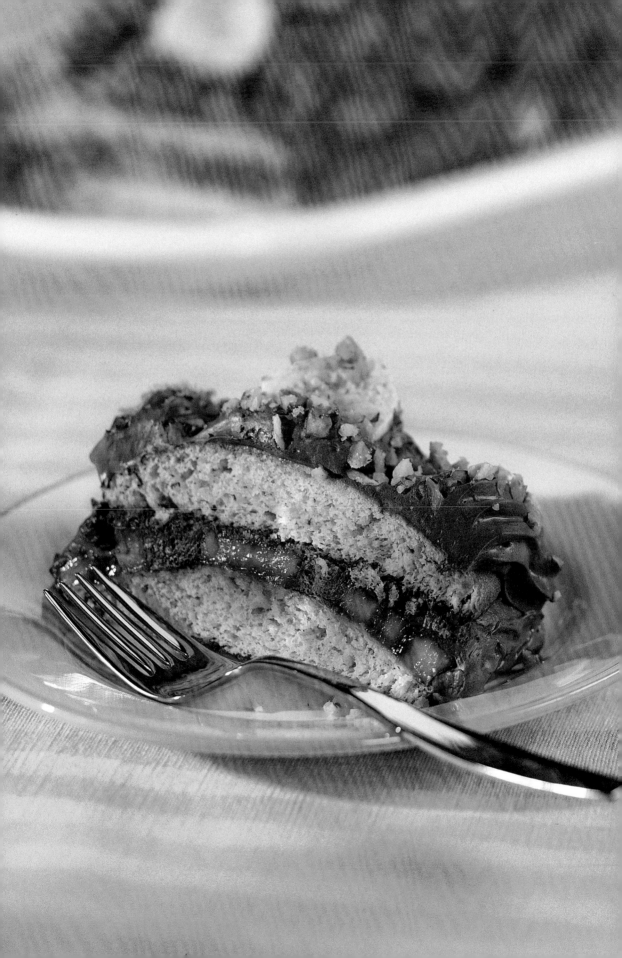

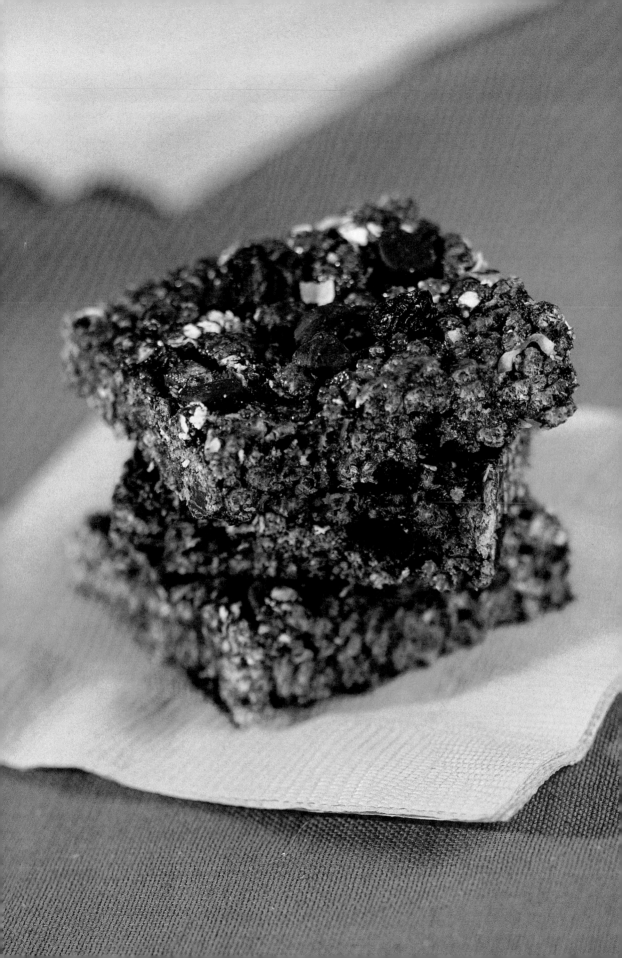

Flying Saucers

- *Baking sheet, lined with waxed paper*

1	package (1 ½ oz/40 g) fat-free instant chocolate pudding mix, sweetened with aspartame	1
1 ½ cups	cold 1% milk	375 mL
1 cup	lower-fat non-dairy whipped topping	250 mL
36	plain chocolate wafers	36

1. In a medium bowl, add chocolate pudding mix to milk. Beat for 2 minutes, until thickened and smooth. Fold in whipped topping.

2. Arrange 18 chocolate wafers in a single layer on prepared cookie sheet. Spoon chocolate pudding mixture onto the wafers. Top with remaining wafers, pressing lightly and smoothing around the edges with a knife, if necessary.

3. Freeze for at least 3 hours, until firm, or in an airtight container for up to 1 month. (If they are too hard to eat, let sit at room temperature for 10 minutes before serving.)

◄ Banana Cream Tiramisu (page 160)

These little ice cream sandwiches are a terrific summertime treat.

Exchanges Per Serving

½ Starch

½ Other Carbohydrate

Nutrient Analysis Per Serving

Calories	74
Protein	2 g
Fat	2 g
Saturated fat	1 g
Carbohydrate	12 g
Fiber	0 g
Cholesterol	2 mg
Sodium	108 mg

This cake looks spectacular with sparklers for a special party.

Tip
If cake is too hard to cut, let stand at room temperature for 10 to 15 minutes before serving.

Ice Cream Fantasy Cake

- *9-inch (23 cm) springform pan*

15	plain chocolate wafers	15
2 tbsp	melted soft margarine	25 mL
4 cups	vanilla ice milk	1 L
	Quick Chocolate Mousse (see recipe, page 157)	
4 cups	raspberry-flavored frozen yogurt	1 L
1 cup	lower-fat non-dairy whipped topping	250 mL
½ cup	calorie-reduced chocolate sundae sauce	50 mL
2 tbsp	chopped peanuts	25 mL
14	strawberries	14

1. In a food processor, grind chocolate wafers into crumbs (or crush them between two sheets of waxed paper with a rolling pin). Mix chocolate crumbs with margarine and press into bottom of springform pan. Refrigerate to cool for 10 to 15 minutes.

2. Let vanilla ice milk soften slightly at room temperature, just until spreadable. Spoon onto chocolate crumb crust and spread evenly. Freeze for 30 minutes, until solid.

3. Spread chocolate mousse over frozen vanilla ice milk. Freeze for 15 minutes, until firm.

4. Scoop frozen yogurt into round balls and arrange over frozen chocolate mousse, covering it completely.

5. Pipe or spoon whipped topping decoratively around the outside edge. Freeze for at least 2 hours or overnight.

6. *To serve:* Drizzle cake top with chocolate sauce, sprinkle with peanuts and garnish with whole strawberries. Remove sides of the springform pan, cut cake into 14 wedges and serve.

Exchanges Per Serving
½ Starch
2 Other Carbohydrate
1 High-Fat Meat

Nutrient Analysis Per Serving

Calories	263
Protein	7 g
Fat	9 g
Saturated fat	4 g
Carbohydrate	41 g
Fiber	0 g
Cholesterol	17 mg
Sodium	194 mg

Raspberry Brownie Parfait

Raspberries and chocolate pair up beautifully in an easy parfait.

6	Chocolate Brownies (see recipe, page 146)	6
2 cups	raspberry-flavored frozen yogurt	500 mL
1/2 cup	fresh raspberries	125 mL
1/4 cup	lower-fat non-dairy whipped topping	50 mL

1. Cut each brownie into small pieces.

2. In each of 4 dessert dishes or parfait glasses, layer 1/4 cup (50 mL) frozen yogurt, 1/8 of the brownie pieces and 1 tbsp (15 mL) fresh raspberries. Repeat layers.

3. Top each parfait with 1 tbsp (15 mL) whipped topping and a "pretty" raspberry.

Dietitian's Message

To lower the carbohydrate/sugar and fat content, you can choose a lower-fat frozen yogurt sweetened with artificial sweetener.

Exchanges Per Serving

1/2	Starch
2 1/2	Other Carbohydrate
1	Medium-Fat Meat
1 1/2	Fat

Nutrient Analysis Per Serving

Calories	320
Protein	8 g
Fat	13 g
Saturated fat	5 g
Carbohydrate	47 g
Fiber	2 g
Cholesterol	53 mg
Sodium	208 mg

Fresh Fruit Parfait

Kids love to make pretty parfaits with their favorite fruit.

Variation

Tropical Parfait:
Use chopped mangoes, papayas and pineapple. Sprinkle 1 tsp (5 mL) toasted shredded coconut on top of each parfait.

2 cups	vanilla ice milk	500 mL
2 cups	fresh fruit (chopped pineapple, chopped kiwi, sliced strawberries, blueberries or sliced oranges)	500 mL
¼ cup	lower-fat non-dairy whipped topping	50 mL

1. In each of 4 dessert dishes or parfait glasses, layer ¼ cup (50 mL) ice milk and ¼ cup (50 mL) fruit. Repeat layers.
2. Top with 1 tbsp (15 mL) whipped topping.

Dietitian's Message *In this case, having dessert ups your nutrient intake. Fruits give us vitamins, antioxidants and fiber, and fresh is always better. Including fresh fruit in an easy dessert recipe such as this one is a delicious way to add another fruit serving to the day.*

Exchanges Per Serving

½	Fruit
½	Other Carbohydrate
½	Medium-Fat Meat

Nutrient Analysis Per Serving

Calories	95
Protein	3 g
Fat	2 g
Saturated fat	1 g
Carbohydrate	19 g
Fiber	2 g
Cholesterol	6 mg
Sodium	36 mg

DESSERTS

Frozen Lemon Pie

- *9-inch (23 cm) pie plate*

I	can (6 oz/175 mL) frozen lemonade concentrate	I
3 cups	vanilla-flavored frozen yogurt	750 mL
I cup	lower-fat sour cream	250 mL
I cup	frozen lower-fat non-dairy whipped topping, divided	250 mL
	Fresh lemon slices, for garnish	

Graham Wafer Crust

¾ cup	graham wafer crumbs	175 mL
3 tbsp	melted soft margarine	45 mL
¼ tsp	ground cinnamon	I mL
¼ tsp	ground nutmeg	I mL

The graham wafer crust is good for many desserts. You can substitute with a store-bought graham wafer crust, but be aware that they are higher in fat and sugar content.

1. Thaw the lemonade concentrate slightly. Put semi-frozen concentrate in a large bowl and beat for 30 seconds. Gradually stir in frozen yogurt. Fold in sour cream and ½ cup (125 mL) of the whipped topping and stir until blended and smooth. Freeze until the mixture will mound on a spoon, about 30 minutes.

2. *Meanwhile, prepare the graham wafer crust:* In a small bowl, combine graham wafer crumbs, margarine, cinnamon and nutmeg. Press into pie plate.

3. Spoon lemonade mixture into prepared piecrust and freeze for at least 4 hours, until firm, or overnight.

4. Cut pie into 8 servings, and garnish each with 1 tbsp (15 mL) whipped topping and lemon slices.

Exchanges Per Serving

½	Starch
2	Other Carbohydrate
I	Medium-Fat Meat
1½	Fat

Nutrient Analysis Per Serving

Calories	265
Protein	5 g
Fat	11 g
Saturated fat	4 g
Carbohydrate	38 g
Fiber	0 g
Cholesterol	10 mg
Sodium	152 mg

Chocolate Bavarian Pie

Chocolate and strawberries are teamed up in this creamy creation.

Tip

You can use a store-bought pie shell for this recipe, or you can make your own: In a small bowl, combine 1½ cups (375 mL) chocolate cookie crumbs with 2 tbsp (25 mL) confectioner's (icing) sugar, sifted, and 6 tbsp (90 mL) melted unsalted butter or margarine. Stir until completely mixed. Distribute evenly in a 9-inch (23 cm) pie plate, pressing firmly against the sides and bottom. Bake at 350°F (180°C) for 10 minutes, until firm. Let cool before filling.

Exchanges Per Serving

1	Starch
1½	Other Carbohydrate
2	Fat

Nutrient Analysis Per Serving

Calories	260
Protein	5 g
Fat	10 g
Saturated fat	3 g
Carbohydrate	40 g
Fiber	1 g
Cholesterol	5 mg
Sodium	219 mg

- *Double boiler*

1½ cups	1% milk, divided	375 mL
1	envelope (¼ oz/7 g) unflavored gelatin	1
⅔ cup	granulated sugar	150 mL
¼ cup	unsweetened cocoa powder, sifted	50 mL
½ tsp	vanilla	2 m
½ cup	plain yogurt	125 mL
	Chocolate cookie crumb pie shell (see tip, at left)	

Strawberry Whipped Topping

½ cup	sliced strawberries, fresh or frozen	125 mL
1 cup	lower-fat non-dairy whipped topping	250 mL

1. Pour 1 cup (250 mL) milk into the top of a double boiler and sprinkle with gelatin; let stand for 2 minutes.

2. In a small bowl, combine granulated sugar and cocoa; whisk into the milk and gelatin mixture. Cook over lightly boiling water, whisking constantly, until thick and smooth, about 10 minutes. Continue to cook, stirring, for 1 minute longer. Remove from heat and stir in the remaining ½ cup (125 mL) milk and vanilla. Let cool to room temperature.

3. Stir in yogurt, cover and refrigerate until mixture begins to set, about 30 minutes.

4. Spoon into chocolate cookie crumb pie shell; chill for at least 4 hours, until set, or overnight.

5. *Prepare the strawberry whipped topping:* If frozen, thaw and drain the berries well; if fresh, wash and pat them dry. In a food processor, purée the berries. Fold into whipped topping. Dollop onto the chilled pie.

Sour Cream and Berry Pie

1	envelope (¼ oz/7 g) unflavored gelatin	1
3 tbsp	cornstarch	45 mL
½ cup	granulated sugar	125 mL
1½ cups	1% milk	375 mL
1 cup	lower-fat sour cream	250 mL
½ cup	plain yogurt	125 mL
1 tsp	vanilla	5 mL
3 cups	mixed raspberries, blueberries, and sliced strawberries	750 mL
	Graham Wafer Crust (see recipe, page 165)	

1. In a medium saucepan, combine gelatin and cornstarch; stir in sugar. Whisk in milk. Cook, stirring, over medium heat until it begins to thicken. Lower heat and allow to simmer, stirring, for 2 minutes longer. Remove from heat and cool slightly.

2. Meanwhile, in a medium bowl, combine sour cream and yogurt. Slowly stir the warm milk mixture into the sour cream mixture and add vanilla. Cover and chill for 1 hour, stirring once or twice, until firm.

3. Wash berries and pat dry with a paper towel. Reserve ½ cup (125 mL) of berries for garnish and fold the rest into the sour cream mixture. Spoon into graham wafer crust and garnish with reserved berries. Cover and chill for 4 to 6 hours, until set.

MAKES 8 SERVINGS

Make this pie in the summer to take advantage of berries at their freshest.

Tip
Before cooking with unflavored gelatin, always allow it to soften in a cold liquid. Gently warm the mixture as the gelatin dissolves. Allowing softened gelatin to boil will destroy its ability to thicken.

Exchanges Per Serving

½	Starch
½	Low-Fat Milk
1	Other Carbohydrate
1	Fat

Nutrient Analysis Per Serving

Calories	215
Protein	5 g
Fat	7 g
Saturated fat	1 g
Carbohydrate	33 g
Fiber	2 g
Cholesterol	2 mg
Sodium	142 mg

You can forgo the pie shell and simply spoon the mousse into dessert bowls or glasses for a different dessert.

Variation

Use your favorite fruit-flavored gelatin and fruit. For example, try orange-flavored gelatin with mandarin oranges or raspberry-flavored gelatin with fresh raspberries.

Exchanges Per Serving

½	Starch
½	Other Carbohydrate
1	Fat

Nutrient Analysis Per Serving

Calories	116
Protein	3 g
Fat	6 g
Saturated fat	1 g
Carbohydrate	13 g
Fiber	1 g
Cholesterol	5 mg
Sodium	151 mg

Strawberry Mousse Pie

1	package (¹/₃ oz/10 g) no-sugar-added strawberry-flavored gelatin	1
²/₃ cup	boiling water	150 mL
	Ice cubes	
½ cup	cold water	125 mL
2 cups	lower-fat non-dairy whipped topping, divided	500 mL
½ cup	plain yogurt	125 mL
1 cup	sliced strawberries, divided	250 mL
	Graham Wafer Crust (see recipe, page 165)	

1. Pour gelatin into a medium bowl and stir in boiling water. Stir for 2 minutes, until all of the gelatin is dissolved.

2. And enough ice to the cold water to make 1 cup (250 mL). Stir into the gelatin until it is slightly thickened and the ice is melted.

3. Stir in 1½ cups (375 mL) of the whipped topping and yogurt and mix until smooth. Fold in ½ cup (125 mL) of the strawberries. Cover and refrigerate for 10 to 14 minutes, or until mixture begins to set.

4. Spoon into graham wafer crust. Refrigerate for 4 hours, or until firm. Garnish with the remaining ½ cup (125 mL) strawberries and the remaining ½ cup (125 mL) whipped topping.

Sweetheart Berry Pie

Top this pretty dessert with pastry shapes, such as stars or Christmas trees, for holiday parties.

- Preheat oven to 450°F (230°C)
- Baking sheet, lined with foil

⅓ cup	granulated sugar, divided	75 mL
1 tsp	ground cinnamon	5 mL
	Pastry for a 9-inch (23 cm) pie (from a mix or homemade)	
1½ cups	blackberries, fresh or frozen	375 mL
1½ cups	raspberries, fresh or frozen	375 mL
1½ cups	blueberries, fresh or frozen	375 mL
1 tbsp	cornstarch	15 mL
3 tbsp	freshly squeezed orange juice	45 mL

1. In a small bowl, combine 1 tsp (5 mL) sugar and cinnamon; set aside.

2. On a lightly floured surface, roll out pastry to ⅛ inch (2.5 mm) thick and cut into 9 heart shapes, using a 3½-inch (8.5 cm) heart-shaped cookie cutter. Sprinkle with cinnamon mixture. Place on prepared baking sheet and bake in preheated oven for 6 to 8 minutes, or until lightly browned. Transfer to a rack and let cool.

3. In a medium saucepan, combine blackberries, raspberries and blueberries. Add the remaining sugar and cornstarch and toss to coat the fruit. Add orange juice. Bring to a boil over medium heat, stirring frequently. Reduce heat to low and simmer for 5 to 10 minutes, until mixture is slightly thickened. Let cool until just warm.

4. Divide berry mixture among 9 individual dessert plates. Top each with a pastry heart.

Dietitian's Message

Blackberries, blueberries and raspberries are rich in antioxidants and fiber. This mouth-watering pie is the perfect dessert for a special festive meal.

Exchanges Per Serving

½	Starch
½	Fruit
½	Other Carbohydrate
1	Fat

Nutrient Analysis Per Serving

Calories	160
Protein	2 g
Fat	6 g
Saturated fat	1 g
Carbohydrate	27 g
Fiber	3 g
Cholesterol	0 mg
Sodium	125 mg

Phyllo Apple Pie

Like Grandma used to make, only better!

Tip

Phyllo pastry dries out very quickly, so work with one sheet at a time, work quickly and keep the roll covered with a damp tea towel.

Variation

Substitute 8 cups (2 L) sliced peaches or pears for the apples.

- Preheat oven to 400°F (200°C)
- 10-inch (25 cm) deep dish pie plate

8	apples (Granny Smith or other cooking variety)	8
1/3 cup	lightly packed brown sugar	75 mL
1/3 cup	granulated sugar	75 mL
1/3 cup	unsweetened apple juice	75 mL
3 tbsp	all-purpose flour	45 mL
2 tbsp	freshly squeezed lemon juice	25 mL
1 tsp	ground cinnamon	5 mL
1/2 tsp	ground ginger	2 mL
1/4 tsp	ground nutmeg	1 mL
4	sheets phyllo pastry	4
1 tbsp	melted butter	15 mL
1 tbsp	additional granulated sugar	15 mL

1. Peel, core and quarter the apples. Cut each quarter into 1/2-inch (1 cm) thick slices and place in a heavy saucepan.

2. In a small bowl, combine brown sugar, granulated sugar, apple juice, flour, lemon juice, cinnamon, ginger and nutmeg. Add to the apples and toss gently to coat. Cover and cook over medium-low heat, stirring occasionally, for 15 to 20 minutes, or until apples are tender. Spoon into pie plate and let cool slightly.

3. Spread out one sheet of phyllo and brush with 1/4 of the butter. Fold one long end over to make a square. Lay another sheet of phyllo crosswise over the first, brush with butter and fold to make a square. Continue layering and buttering the phyllo sheets, but don't butter the top one. Place the phyllo stack on the pie filling. Dot with the remaining butter and sprinkle lightly with 1 tbsp (15 mL) granulated sugar.

4. Gather the edges of the phyllo to form a ruffle around the pie. Spray the ruffle with vegetable spray. Cut slits into the phyllo top to allow steam to escape.

5. Bake in preheated oven for 15 minutes, until phyllo is golden.

Exchanges Per Serving

1	Starch
1	Fruit
1	Other Carbohydrate
1/2	Fat

Nutrient Analysis Per Serving

Calories	198
Protein	1 g
Fat	3 g
Saturated fat	1 g
Carbohydrate	45 g
Fiber	3 g
Cholesterol	4 mg
Sodium	61 mg

Peanut Butter Apple Crisp

Peanut butter chips add a surprise twist to a traditional dessert.

- Preheat oven to 350°F (180°C)
- 9-inch (2.5 L) square glass baking pan, sprayed with vegetable spray

Fruit Layer

4 cups	peeled and sliced apples	1 L
1/3 cup	peanut butter chips	75 mL
1/4 cup	granulated sugar	50 mL
2 tbsp	all-purpose flour	25 mL

Topping

1 cup	quick-cooking rolled oats	250 mL
1/3 cup	all-purpose flour	75 mL
1/3 cup	lightly packed brown sugar	75 mL
1/4 cup	soft margarine	50 mL
1/2 tsp	ground cinnamon	2 mL

1. *Prepare the fruit layer:* In a large bowl, stir together apples, peanut butter chips, sugar and flour. Spread into prepared pan.

2. *Prepare the topping:* In a medium bowl, combine oats, flour, brown sugar, margarine and cinnamon until crumbly. Sprinkle over the apple layer.

3. Bake in preheated oven for 40 to 45 minutes, or until apples are tender. Cut into 9 squares and serve warm.

Dietitian's Message
The addition of peanut butter chips to this recipe makes it very kid-friendly. And it's a way to sneak in some fruit!

Tips

Read the labels on peanut butter chips. Some have twice as many grams of fat as others. Choose the lower-fat version when possible.

Metal pans can discolor when fruit is baked in them, so always use a tempered glass baking dish for fruit desserts.

Exchanges Per Serving

1	Starch
1/2	Fruit
1	Other Carbohydrate
2	Fat

Nutrient Analysis Per Serving

Calories	247
Protein	3 g
Fat	10 g
Saturated fat	3 g
Carbohydrate	40 g
Fiber	3 g
Cholesterol	0 mg
Sodium	69 mg

You can use any apples for this recipe, but baking apples, such as Granny Smith, Northern Spy or Crispin, retain their shape better and tend to be more tart, which is a delicious contrast to the sweet filling.

Tips

You can use homemade Fruity Granola (see recipe, page 41) or buy lower-fat granola at the supermarket.

To serve leftover baked apples for breakfast, place on a microwave-safe dessert dish and microwave on Medium-High (70%) for about 1 to 1½ minutes.

Exchanges Per Serving

½	Starch
1½	Fruit
1½	Fat

Nutrient Analysis Per Serving

Calories	198
Protein	2 g
Fat	7 g
Saturated fat	3 g
Carbohydrate	35 g
Fiber	4 g
Cholesterol	10 mg
Sodium	48 mg

172

Baked Apples with Granola

- Preheat oven to 375°F (190°C)
- 8-inch (2 L) square glass baking dish

4	baking apples	4
⅓ cup	lower-fat granola	75 mL
2 tbsp	raisins	25 mL
2 tbsp	slivered almonds	25 mL
4 tsp	butter	20 mL
1 tsp	ground cinnamon	5 mL
¼ cup	unsweetened apple juice	50 mL

1. Core apples without cutting through the base of the apple and remove the core. Peel a ¾-inch (2 cm) strip around the top of each apple. Place in the baking dish.

2. In a small bowl, combine granola, raisins and almonds. Stuff into apple cavities.

3. Dot 1 tsp (5 mL) butter on top of the filling in each apple and sprinkle with cinnamon. Pour apple juice over the apples.

4. Bake in preheated oven, basting often with apple juice, for 50 minutes to 1 hour, or until apples are very tender. Let cool slightly before serving warm.

Dietitian's Message *Cereal with fruit is a good way to start the day, so try serving this dessert for breakfast! This dish is packed with energy and nutrients. In addition, apples contain pectin, a soluble fiber that gives it a lower glycemic index.*

Cherry Cobbler

- Preheat oven to 375°F (190°C)
- 9-inch (2.5 L) square baking dish, sprayed with vegetable spray

Filling

¼ cup	granulated sugar	50 mL
1 tbsp	cornstarch	15 mL
3 cups	pitted sweet cherries	750 mL

Topping

½ cup	all-purpose flour	125 mL
¼ cup	granulated sugar	50 mL
½ tsp	baking powder	2 mL
¼ tsp	salt	1 mL
1	large egg	1
1 tbsp	soft margarine	15 mL
1 tbsp	1% milk	15 mL
1 tbsp	granulated sugar	15 mL
½ tsp	ground cinnamon	2 mL

1. *Prepare the filling:* In a medium saucepan, combine sugar and cornstarch and toss with cherries. Add ¼ cup (50 mL) water and stir to mix. Bring to a boil over medium heat, stirring frequently. Simmer for 5 minutes, until slightly thickened.

2. *Prepare the topping:* In a small bowl, combine flour, sugar, baking powder and salt. In another small bowl, using an electric mixer, beat egg and margarine; add milk. Beat in flour mixture until smooth.

3. Spread hot fruit in prepared baking dish and drop batter by heaping tablespoonfuls (15 mL) evenly over top.

4. In a small bowl, combine sugar and cinnamon; sprinkle over topping.

5. Bake in preheated oven for 25 to 30 minutes, or until browned.

This old-fashioned dessert is yummy served with vanilla frozen yogurt or ice milk, but keep in mind that these will increase the carbohydrate.

Variation

Substitute your favorite seasonal fruit for the cherries. Try blueberries, blackberries, sliced plums, sliced apricots or sliced peaches.

Exchanges Per Serving

½	Starch
1	Fruit
1	Other Carbohydrate
½	Fat

Nutrient Analysis Per Serving

Calories	191
Protein	3 g
Fat	4 g
Saturated fat	1 g
Carbohydrate	38 g
Fiber	1 g
Cholesterol	36 mg
Sodium	148 mg

Angel Tunnel Cake

An angel food cake mix is a good low-fat base for many imaginative desserts. This cake, with its surprise filling, will wow your family and guests.

Tip

It's hard to cut an angel food cake because it is sticky. Try using a wet knife with a serrated edge, and use your fingers to help hollow out the trench.

1	prepared vanilla or chocolate angel food cake (from mix, store-bought or homemade)	1
1	package (1½ oz/40 g) fat-free instant chocolate pudding mix, sweetened with aspartame	1
1½ cups	1% milk	375 mL
3 cups	lower-fat non-dairy whipped topping, divided	750 mL
2 tbsp	unsweetened cocoa powder	25 mL

1. Slice a 1-inch (2.5 cm) layer off the top of the cake. Gently hollow out a trench 1½ inches (4 cm) wide and 2 inches (5 cm) deep from the bottom piece. Cut the cake removed from the trench into small pieces.

2. In a large bowl, beat pudding mix and milk for 2 minutes, until thickened and smooth. Stir in 1 cup (250 mL) of the whipped topping and the reserved cake pieces. Fill the trench with the pudding mixture and replace the top of the cake.

3. In a medium bowl, sift cocoa into the remaining 2 cups (500 mL) whipped topping and stir gently until smooth. Frost cake with chocolate whipped topping and chill for at least 4 hours, until set, or overnight.

Dietitian's Message *Angel food cake is low in calories because it is made primarily with egg whites.*

Exchanges Per Serving

1	Starch
1½	Other Carbohydrate

Nutrient Analysis Per Serving

Calories	171
Protein	5 g
Fat	2 g
Saturated fat	1 g
Carbohydrate	36 g
Fiber	0 g
Cholesterol	6 mg
Sodium	268 mg

Fruit-Filled Angel Tunnel Cake

Angel tunnel cakes are easier than they look when you use a cake mix!

1	prepared vanilla or lemon angel food cake (from mix, store-bought or homemade)	1
1	package (1⅓ oz/38 g) calorie-reduced vanilla mousse mix	1
1½ cups	1% milk	375 mL
2 cups	lower-fat non-dairy whipped topping, divided	500 mL
1 cup	diced fresh fruit (such as strawberries, blueberries, kiwi)	250 mL
1 tbsp	grated lemon zest	15 mL

1. Slice a 1-inch (2.5 cm) layer off the top of the cake. Gently hollow out a trench 1½ inches (4 cm) wide and 2 inches (5 cm) deep from the bottom piece. Cut the cake removed from the trench into small pieces.

2. In a medium bowl, beat vanilla mousse mix and milk for 3 minutes, until thickened. Fold in ½ cup (125 mL) of the whipped topping, fresh fruit, lemon zest and cake pieces. Fill the trench with the fruit mixture and replace the top of the cake.

3. Frost with the remaining 1½ cups (375 mL) whipped topping and chill for at least 4 hours, until set, or overnight. Garnish with lemon slices just before serving.

Exchanges Per Serving

1	Starch
1	Other Carbohydrate

Nutrient Analysis Per Serving

Calories	164
Protein	5 g
Fat	1 g
Saturated fat	1 g
Carbohydrate	35 g
Fiber	0 g
Cholesterol	4 mg
Sodium	263 mg

The cran-apple topping makes this a light and festive dessert to serve at Christmastime.

Tip

Because heat rises, oven temperatures are not even throughout. For best results, bake cakes in the very center of the oven. If baking more than one item at a time, stagger them on the same rack so they don't touch the walls of the oven or each other.

Exchanges Per Serving

½ Starch

½ Fruit

1 Other Carbohydrate

Nutrient Analysis Per Serving

Calories	143
Protein	2 g
Fat	0 g
Saturated fat	0 g
Carbohydrate	34 g
Fiber	1 g
Cholesterol	0 mg
Sodium	182 mg

Spiced Angel Food Cake

- Preheat oven to 325°F (160°C)
- 10-inch (4 L) tube pan, ungreased

1	package (1 lb/450 g) vanilla angel food cake mix	1
1 tsp	ground cinnamon	5 mL
1 tsp	ground ginger	5 mL
½ tsp	ground nutmeg	2 mL

Cran-apple Topping

4	red apples (e.g., Macintosh), cored and thinly sliced	4
½ cup	freshly squeezed orange juice	125 mL
⅓ cup	lightly packed brown sugar	75 mL
2 tsp	cornstarch	10 mL
1 tsp	ground cinnamon	5 mL
1 cup	cranberries, fresh or frozen	250 mL

1. To the dry cake mix, add cinnamon, ginger and nutmeg, then bake according to package instructions. Let cool in the pan, inverted on a wire rack.

2. *Prepare the cran-apple topping:* Put apples in a large skillet. In a small bowl, stir together orange juice, brown sugar and cornstarch until smooth. Add cinnamon and ¼ cup (50 mL) water. Pour orange juice mixture over the apples and cook over medium heat, stirring occasionally, for 5 to 8 minutes, until juice starts to bubble. Reduce heat to low and add cranberries; simmer for 10 to 15 minutes, or until berries pop.

3. Serve the warm topping over slices of cake.

Striped Strawberry Cake

- Preheat oven to 350°F (180°C)
- 13- by 9-inch (3 L) baking pan, sprayed with vegetable spray

1	package (18¼ oz/515 g) white cake mix	1
1	package (⅓ oz/10 g) no-sugar-added strawberry-flavored gelatin	1
1 cup	boiling water	250 mL
½ cup	cold water	125 mL
2 cups	lower-fat non-dairy whipped topping	500 mL
20	strawberries	20

1. Bake the cake in the prepared pan according to package instructions. Let cool in the pan for 10 minutes. Remove from the pan and let cool completely on a rack. Wash the pan.

2. In a medium bowl, dissolve gelatin in boiling water. Add cold water and let gelatin cool to room temperature, but do not let it begin to set.

3. When cake is cool, return it to the clean pan and prick it with a large serving fork at ½-inch (1 cm) intervals.

4. Pour cooled gelatin evenly over the cake, cover and refrigerate for 3 to 4 hours, until gelatin is set.

5. Dip the pan in warm water, invert onto a serving plate and remove the pan.

6. Frost the top and sides of the cake with whipped topping. Mark 20 even pieces in the frosting and garnish each square with a sliced and fanned strawberry.

Cakes with gelatin stripes have been a birthday party favorite for years. Now you can make a cake that's low in sugar and fat by using sugar-free gelatin and lower-fat whipped topping.

Variation

Make seasonal striped cakes: pink hearts for Valentine's Day; green trees for Christmas. Use a shaped cake pan and gelatin that is the appropriate color, and add food coloring to the whipped topping.

Exchanges Per Serving

½ Starch

1 Other Carbohydrate

½ Fat

Nutrient Analysis Per Serving

Calories	130
Protein	2 g
Fat	3 g
Saturated fat	1 g
Carbohydrate	23 g
Fiber	0 g
Cholesterol	2 mg
Sodium	185 mg

*Candy and chocolate
topping make plain
cupcakes into
a special treat
for parties!*

Tip

As a general rule, cake
and muffin batter
should fill a pan about
2/3 full. If you don't fill
pans enough, your
cakes will be flat; if
you fill them too
much, they will
overflow and make
a mess!

Peppermint Angel Cupcakes

- *Preheat oven to 350°F (180°C)*
- *24 muffin cups, lined with paper liners*

½ cup	red, green and white peppermint candies	125 mL
I	package (1 lb/450 g) white angel food cake mix	I
½ cup	Chocolate Sauce (see recipe, page 159)	125 mL

1. Crush candies in a food processor or by placing them between tea towels or in a resealable freezer bag and smashing them with a hammer.

2. Prepare cake batter according to package instructions, then stir in ½ of the crushed candies. Pour into prepared muffin cups.

3. Bake in preheated oven for 30 minutes, rotating pans halfway, until tops are golden and firm. Immediately remove from the pan to cool on a rack.

4. Drizzle chocolate sauce on top of the cupcakes and sprinkle with the remaining candies.

**Exchanges
Per Serving**

½   Starch

I   Other
Carbohydrate

**Nutrient Analysis
Per Serving**

Calories	103
Protein	2 g
Fat	0 g
Saturated fat	0 g
Carbohydrate	25 g
Fiber	0 g
Cholesterol	0 mg
Sodium	129 mg

Spicy Apple Cupcakes

- Preheat oven to 350°F (180°C)
- 10 muffin cups, lined with paper cups or sprayed with vegetable spray

1 cup	all-purpose flour	250 mL
1 tsp	pumpkin pie spice	5 mL
½ tsp	baking powder	2 mL
½ tsp	baking soda	2 mL
½ tsp	salt	2 mL
½ cup	granulated sugar	125 mL
¼ cup	lightly packed brown sugar	50 mL
¼ cup	soft margarine	50 mL
1	large egg	1
½ tsp	vanilla	2 mL
½ cup	unsweetened applesauce	125 mL

The applesauce in the batter serves as a partial substitute for fat and sugar, while keeping the cupcakes moist and flavorful.

Variation

If you wish, mix a simple glaze of ½ cup (125 mL) confectioner's (icing) sugar, sifted, and 2 tbsp (25 mL) water or unsweetened apple juice to drizzle on these cupcakes.

1. In a small bowl, combine flour, pumpkin pie spice, baking powder, baking soda and salt.

2. In a medium bowl, using an electric mixer or wooden spoon, cream granulated sugar, brown sugar and margarine until fluffy. Beat in egg and vanilla. Stir in flour mixture until blended. Stir in applesauce.

3. Divide batter among the muffin tins, filling them ½ full. Bake in preheated oven for 20 to 25 minutes, or until a toothpick inserted in the center comes out clean. Let cool in pan on a rack for 10 minutes. Transfer to rack to cool completely.

Exchanges Per Serving

½	Starch
1	Other Carbohydrate
1	Fat

Nutrient Analysis Per Serving

Calories	160
Protein	2 g
Fat	5 g
Saturated fat	1 g
Carbohydrate	27 g
Fiber	1 g
Cholesterol	22 mg
Sodium	189 mg

Library and Archives Canada Cataloguing in Publication

Bartley, Colleen, 1953–
America's best cookbook for kids with diabetes / Colleen Bartley.

Includes index.
ISBN 0-7788-0116-0

1. Diabetes in children — Diet therapy — Recipes. I. Title.

RC662.B364 2005   641.5'6314   C2004-906535-1

Index

tomatoes, fresh
  BLT Wraps, 87
  Chicken Caesar Wraps, 86
  Chicken Fajita Salad, 75
  French Bread Pizza, 101
  Guacamole Nachos, 60
  Hot Dog Kabobs, 94
  Pasta Salad on a Stick, 72
  Picnic Hero, 90
  ripening, 90
  Salad Bar Subs, 92
  Salsa and Tortilla Chips, 58
  Soft Chicken Tacos, 116
  Surprise Quick Quiche (variation), 28
  Taco Salad, 73
  Tex's Tacos, 117
  Tuna Egg Salad Subs, 93
  Zucchini Boats, 84
tortilla chips
  Salsa and Tortilla Chips, 58
  Taco Salad, 73
tortillas
  BLT Wraps, 87
  Breakfast Quesadillas, 42
  Chicken Caesar Wraps, 86
  Chicken Fajita Salad, 75
  Garden Burritos, 118
  Guacamole Nachos, 60
  Mexican Scrambled Eggs, 27
  Quick Quesadillas, 61
  Refrito Quesadillas, 120
  Salsa and Tortilla Chips, 58
  Soft Chicken Tacos, 116
tuna
  Chicken Salad Nests (variation), 74
  Tuna Burgers, 100
  Tuna Egg Salad Subs, 93
  Tuna Melts on Pitas, 89
Tuna Burgers, 100
Tuna Egg Salad Subs, 93
Tuna Melts on Pitas, 89
turkey
  Garden Burritos (variation), 118
  Hawaiian Chili, 121
  Homemade Turkey Sausage, 39
  Lasagna, 122
  Lazy Lasagna, 124
  Open-Face Deli Melts, 88
  Pasta Salad on a Stick, 72
  Picnic Hero, 90
  Spicy Mini Meatloaves, 134
  Taco Pizza, 104

Taco Salad, 73
Tex's Tacos, 117
Turkey-Mozza Burgers, 95
Turkey-Mozza Burgers, 95
Turkey Sausage, Homemade, 39

V
Valentine's Day dishes
  Salmon Croquettes (variation), 111
  Striped Strawberry Cake (variation), 177
  Sweetheart Berry Pie, 169
vegetables, 77–84. *See also specific types of vegetables*
vegetarian dishes. *See* meatless dishes
Virtuous Veggie Pizza, 106

W
waffles, 30, 37
walnuts
  Banana Bread, 152
  Banana Cream Tiramisu, 160
  Chocolate Brownies, 146
water chestnuts
  Teriyaki Burgers, 96
websites, 10, 15, 16, 17, 22
wheat germ
  Blender Breakfast Blast, 44
  Fruity Granola, 41
  Peanut Butter Muffins, 150
whipped topping
  Angel Tunnel Cake, 174
  Banana Cream Tiramisu, 160
  Chocolate and Strawberry Waffles, 37
  Chocolate Bavarian Pie, 166
  Crunchy French Toast, 38
  Flying Saucers, 161
  Fresh Fruit Parfait, 164
  Frozen Lemon Pie, 165
  Fruit-Filled Angel Tunnel Cake, 175
  Fruit on a Cloud, 155
  Ice Cream Fantasy Cake, 162
  Quick Chocolate Mousse, 157
  Raspberry Brownie Parfait, 163
  Rocky Road Mousse, 158
  Strawberry Mousse Pie, 168
  Striped Strawberry Cake, 177
wieners
  Chili Burgers (variation), 97
  Hot Dog Kabobs, 94

Y

yogurt
- Blender Breakfast Blast, 44
- Chocolate Bavarian Pie, 166
- Creamy Dreamy Fruit Salad, 156
- Hummus and Pita Chips, 57
- Ice Cream Fantasy Cake, 162
- Light Tartar Sauce, 99
- Pancake or Waffle Batter, 30
- Peanut Butter Muffins, 150
- Potato Chip Fish, 109
- Rocky Road Mousse, 158
- Smashed Potatoes, 77

Sour Cream and Berry Pie, 167
Strawberry Mousse Pie, 168
yogurt, frozen. *See also* ice cream/ice milk
- Frozen Lemon Pie, 165
- Pancake Banana Splits, 34
- Peach Melba Smoothie, 45
- Raspberry Brownie Parfait, 163

Z

zucchini
- Virtuous Veggie Pizza, 106
- Zucchini Boats, 84
Zucchini Boats, 84

Also Available
from Robert Rose

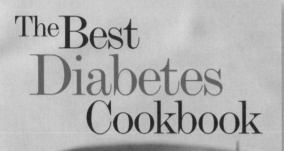

The Best
Diabetes
Cookbook

Edited by
KATHERINE E. YOUNKER
MBA, RD, Certified Diabetes Educator

America's Everyday
Diabetes
Cookbook

Edited by
Katherine E. Younker
MBA, RD, Certified Diabetes Educator

Robert
ROSE